# *Desperate* HOPE

## EXPERIENCING GOD IN THE MIDST OF BREAST CANCER

## BARBARA MILLIGAN

InterVarsity Press
Downers Grove, Illinois

138229

*InterVarsity Press*
*P.O. Box 1400, Downers Grove, IL 60515*
*World Wide Web: www.ivpress.com*
*E-mail: mail@ivpress.com*

*InterVarsity Press® is the book-publishing division of InterVarsity Christian Fellowship/USA®, a student movement active on campus at hundreds of universities, colleges and schools of nursing in the United States of America, and a member movement of the International Fellowship of Evangelical Students. For information about local and regional activities, write Public Relations Dept., InterVarsity Christian Fellowship/USA, 6400 Schroeder Rd., P.O. Box 7895, Madison, WI 53707-7895.*

*All Scripture quotations, unless otherwise indicated, are taken from the* Holy Bible, New International Version.® NIV®. *Copyright ©1973, 1978, 1984 by International Bible Society. Used by permission of Zondervan Publishing House. All rights reserved.*

*Cover photograph: SuperStock*

*ISBN 0-8308-1924-X*

*Printed in the United States of America* ♾

**Library of Congress Cataloging-in-Publication Data**

*Milligan, Barbara, 1949-*
   *Desperate hope: experiencing God in the midst of breast cancer/*
*Barbara Milligan.*
      *p.   cm.*
   *Includes bibliographical references (p.      ).*
   *ISBN 0-8308-1924-X (pbk.: alk. paper)*
   *1. Breast—Cancer—Patients—Religious life.   I. Title.*
*BV4910.33.M55   1999*
*248.8'619699449—dc21*
                                                                                99-34661
                                                                                   *CIP*

| 20 | 19 | 18 | 17 | 16 | 15 | 14 | 13 | 12 | 11 | 10 | 9 | 8 | 7 | 6 | 5 | 4 | 3 | 2 | 1 |
|----|----|----|----|----|----|----|----|----|----|----|---|---|---|---|---|---|---|---|---|
| 16 | 15 | 14 | 13 | 12 | 11 | 10 | 09 | 08 | 07 | 06 | 05 | 04 | 03 | 02 | 01 | 00 | 99 | | |

*For my husband, John*

*And in memory of Karen Rae Mahaffey Notor,*
*Margo ("Margaret") Underwood, Joan Van Kampen*
*and Sarah Markam, who are now experiencing God face to face*

# CONTENTS

## Acknowledgments

Writing a book and having breast cancer are alike in one way: you can't survive without the support of friends. I am deeply grateful to those named here and to the many other friends who encouraged me or prayed for me while I worked on this book.

Lonnie Hull Dupont, Steven H. Behrends, M.D., John Boykin, Timothy Jones, Francis Heatherley and Jan M. Johnson provided invaluable professional advice. Also, Victoria Case, Sharon N. Jones, Lisa Largent, Arda Rooks, Anna Sider and Sally E. Stuart helped me locate potential interviewees. A special thanks goes to my editor at InterVarsity Press, Cynthia Bunch-Hotaling, for her helpful suggestions and guidance, and to the IVP staff for their support. I also appreciate the encouragement I've received from my parents, William and Pauline Malacarne; from Cecil, Dana, Heather and Lauren Malacarne; and from Jane Hudkins and Susan O'Hair. For practical help, I want to thank Pastor John Shafe, Rachel Behrends, Jane Stone, David Talbott and two nurses at the Palo Alto Medical Foundation—Rosemary Maresca, R.N., and June Ghahraman, R.N. And for early inspiration that gave me confidence nearly three decades later, I owe many thanks to John Sider, Richard Morrow and Carole Fuester.

This book would not exist without the sixteen women and three men who shared their stories with me. I am forever indebted to these special friends for pouring out their souls to the total stranger that I was to most of them at first. They continually encouraged me through their prayers, messages and enthusiasm. I also appreciate the generous support I received from their families.

My friend Juanita Ryan helped me in ways too numerous to name—everything from reviewing several revisions of the same chapters to picking me up off the emotional pavement. I don't know what I would have done without her. I am deeply grateful also to Maria and Pete Sommer, Rose Marie Springer, Joyce Landorf Heatherley, Kathy Ley and my writers critique group—Cathleen Armstrong, Normajean Hinders, Laurie Kehler, Pat Sikora, Judy Squier and Deby Turnrose—for their feedback on the manuscript, their prayers and their affirmation. And I appreciate the encouragement of my cancer support group, Women Together Living with Cancer.

I owe thousands of hours of cooking, grocery shopping and house-cleaning to my husband, John Milligan, who never let me feel guilty for not doing my fair share after I began writing this book. But more important, I would not have attempted this project without his shared vision, his expressed confidence in me, his continual prayers for me and his many useful suggestions for reorganizing or rewriting the text. Along with my other friends, he demonstrates for me every day the extravagance of God's love.

Finally, I thank my God, who coached me, comforted me, dropped extraordinary opportunities into my lap and every day gave me reasons to keep working. For me, this book has begun a new series of wildly wonderful adventures in experiencing the God of my own desperate hope.

# 1

## TURNING TO THE GOD OF OUR DESPERATE HOPE

More out of politeness than genuine interest, I slowly turned the pages of the most bizarre photo album I'd ever seen: page after page of naked women—most of them middle-aged and sagging—shown only from the neck to the waist. Each "before" shot showed a breast on one side of the woman and only a thin diagonal or horizontal scar on the other side. The matching "after" shot showed the same woman with two almost matching breasts. *I guess it's an improvement,* I told myself.

But my mind was in a fog. I thought I heard the nurse, in whose office I was sitting, exclaim about what "wonderful reconstructive surgery they're doing these days." As I watched her lips move, a few of her phrases droned in my ears like a radio commercial: "could stretch some of your chest muscles," "borrow some skin from your leg," "tattoo a 'nipple' and even darken it. . . ."

*I'm dreaming,* I thought to myself. *This photo album isn't real, this nurse and my husband sitting next to me aren't real, and breast cancer is what happens to other women, not to me.*

Every couple of minutes I tried to mentally peer through the fog and ask myself what I was feeling. But all I could tell was that I felt either nothing or everything. However, it didn't seem to matter. I wasn't sure what mattered any more.

Only a few hours earlier, my husband, John, and I had been told by my surgeon that the breast tissue he had biopsied because of an "atypical" mammogram contained a malignant tumor. Almost within the same breath, he had told me that he recommended a mastectomy, rather than a lumpectomy and radiation, because of the small size of my breast and the central location of the tumor.

*I have breast cancer,* I thought. *And I may have to lose my entire breast. But I feel perfectly healthy.*

The next thing I knew, John and I were scheduling an appointment for that afternoon with the briefing nurse, who would talk to us about reconstructive surgery and show us the grotesque photos. Sometime between those two appointments, I remember sitting in our car, crying, with my head on John's shoulder and his hands stroking my back.

## Questioning God

At home that evening I was dismayed to realize that I hadn't prayed since hearing the diagnosis. A practice that for most of my life had seemed as natural as breathing was gone, and I had no idea why. God had always proven himself good and loving and trustworthy to me. I loved him, and I knew I needed him desperately—especially now. But I felt distant from him.

*Dear God, help me to talk to you.* The words finally formed a coherent sentence in my mind.

The next morning, as I sat quietly, trying to slow my spinning head and see through the residual fog, God answered that simple prayer. As I cried out to him, I was surprised to find some questions—some of which I'd never asked before—spilling out of the deepest corners of my heart. They went something like this:

Are you still there, Lord? Why did you let this happen? I don't believe you're punishing me, but did I do something to cause this cancer in my body? Should I have exercised five times a week instead of four? Should I have eaten *more* broccoli and spinach? Am I hiding some stress so effectively that I'm not aware of it? Could you possibly have forgotten about me for a moment—just long enough that some cancer cells sneaked into my body? Do I really have to lose my breast? Will the cancer keep coming back and eventually kill me? Do you have a *purpose* for me in all this?

Crying out to God with those questions was one of the best things I've ever done. Over the next several weeks as I persisted in my questioning, I sensed his presence and more of his tender love toward me. I also realized that he had heard those and similar questions before, from many other women: Why is this happening? Have you abandoned me? Are you punishing me? Did I do something to cause my cancer? Am I going to die? Are you displeased because I'm afraid? Why don't my friends understand me? Why me? And, Why is this happening to me?

I know absolutely that God is not disturbed by such questions. He handles "worse" questions, in his typically merciful ways, every day. I also know that he wants to respond to each of us—not always by answering our specific questions but by giving us what we most want, perhaps unknowingly, in the first place: his presence and his love.

### Facing the Emotions

Although my experience with cancer ended, medically speaking, only two months after it began, my life was forever changed. During that time and for several months afterward, I felt the full range of emotions that normally accompany a trauma: shock, fear, grief, anger, frustration and guilt feelings. Of course, I didn't deal with each emotion once and then lay it to rest. In twos or threes, and sometimes all at once, they kept returning, just like the ants I always thought I'd gotten rid of in my bathroom.

In looking back, I see that the experience of shock, fear, grief, anger, and so on is no longer for myself alone. It's for Sarah, who had to tell her young children that she might die sooner rather than later. It's for Joan, whose cancer has reached her brain, blurring her vision and making her dizzy. It's for twenty-one-year-old Janaha and for many daughters and sons like her, who felt alone and helpless as they watched their mothers die. It's for the twenty women in this country who were diagnosed with breast cancer in the past hour.[1] It's for the nearly forty-four thousand women in the United States who will die of breast cancer this year.[2] And it's for everyone who fears this disease for which there is no known prevention and no known cure.

I've heard some Christians say, "But all things work together for *good.* God can *take away* the shock, the fear and all your other negative feelings." Yes, he can. But if he did, many of us wouldn't have the compassion, the *passion,* that we have experienced about life and about God and about those we love. As long as God hates evil—including the evil of breast cancer—shouldn't *we* hate evil? As long as God grieves, shouldn't *we* grieve? When we experience these "negative" feelings and tell God about them, we can experience more of God. We also give God the opportunity to respond to our feelings. When we tell him we're afraid, we can receive his comfort. When we tell him we're angry, he can show us why we're angry and how to respond to the causes of our anger. When we grieve, he grieves with us and helps us to fully understand the value of our loss. He is a *feeling* God—a God who reveals more of himself to us as we experience what he is already feeling.

## Using This Book

I am only one of thousands of women who have experienced God in the midst of breast cancer. In this book you will meet fifteen others who had or who still have breast cancer. In addition, you will meet the husbands of two of them, and the husband of my friend Karen, who died of breast cancer at age thirty-three.. You will also meet Janaha (pronounced Juh-NAY-uh), mentioned earlier, who as a teenager provided care for her mother, who was dying of breast cancer.

All of these women and men are followers of Christ, but their backgrounds are otherwise varied: the women's ages at the time of diagnosis range from thirty-six to sixty-five; they're both single and married; they represent many vocations; their church backgrounds include Roman Catholic, Eastern Orthodox and many Protestant denominations; their ethnic backgrounds are rooted in Africa, Asia, Latin America and Europe (and three of them are not American citizens); except for Joan, a Canadian, they live in a variety of cities and towns throughout the western United States. They all have unique stories to tell of how they experienced God in the midst of breast cancer and how he replaced some of their deepest fears with hope.

This book is not only for women who have been diagnosed with breast cancer. It's also for their husbands, their sons and daughters, their parents, their sisters and brothers, their friends, their pastors and church leaders, their health care professionals, their employers and coworkers, and anyone else who wants to know how to respond to a woman who has breast cancer. Although a small percentage of men get breast cancer, this book addresses the separate issues that women face, as well as the issues faced by both women and men.

The chapters are arranged in a sequence that corresponds to the approximate order in which the issues discussed tend to occur in a woman's experience of breast cancer. Some chapters include sidebars that offer convenient reference lists of suggestions that might help you, whether you have breast cancer yourself or you are a friend or family member of someone who has breast cancer.

At the end of the book you'll find three appendixes that address specific topics. If you have breast cancer yourself, you'll find some suggestions on how to find spiritual support, including a support group or a network of others who have had breast cancer. If you are the husband of a woman who has breast cancer, you'll find some concrete ways that you can help your wife regain her sense of sexuality. If you are a friend or a family member, you'll find many suggestions for helping her practically, emotionally and spiritually. A fourth appendix lists some resources that may help you whether you have cancer yourself or want only to understand the issues related to having cancer.

You may wonder why I use the editorial *we* throughout the book, as if I've personally experienced nearly everything that can happen to a woman who has breast cancer. For the record, I had a drive-thru mastectomy, in which I was sent home two hours after the surgery. I had no follow-up treatment—no chemotherapy, no radiation, no tamoxifen, no alternative or experimental therapy. Nor do I have children, even though I often refer to "our children." I use "we" in the text as a way of identifying with the people I interviewed and perhaps with you, the reader.

The experience of having breast cancer never ends, even if the cancer does. Although I was pronounced cured, I still face the cancer that is no longer there. I face it every time I take off my clothes and look down at my chest. I face it every time I have sensations of breast tenderness on my left side and then realize that my nerve endings—the ones that are still alive—are fooling me once again. I face it every time I lay my remaining breast on the cold slab of the mammography machine, and then again as I wait vigilantly for the results. I face it every time another friend hears the word *malignant* from her doctor. And I face it every time it kills another friend.

Yet, for all of us whose stories are told in this book, facing the enemy of breast cancer has been a journey of desperate hope—not because there's anything good about the disease, but because we have experienced God in the midst of it. Rachel remembers "desperately" needing to know that God was with her. Judy remembers feeling that she was hanging over a cliff but was being held by the firm grasp of God. And Bonita remembers feeling "absolutely desperate for hope." Our God, whose power is far greater than all the evils in the world combined, has promised to be with us, to comfort us and to help us throughout our experience of breast cancer.

This book is not intended either as a scientific study or as an exhaustive resource—medically, emotionally, interrelationally or even spiritually. Many excellent resources already exist that offer information about the disease and its related issues. This book is intended, however, as a testament that we have a God who hears the questioning cries of our hearts and who responds out of his infinite love for us, so that we can experience his love, even while we have breast cancer. For it is only by that love that our desperate hope is fulfilled.

Whether you have—or did have—breast cancer yourself or you know someone who does, may these pages help you to personally experience the God of our desperate hope.

# 2

## RESPONDING TO FEELINGS OF FEAR, ANXIETY & SADNESS

When we've been diagnosed with breast cancer, we face an avalanche of feelings. We may feel like young children who need to be held and comforted by a loving parent. We begin to grasp how fragile our lives are. And we may become more aware of how much we need God. Yet, at a time that we need God most, we may find it difficult to turn to him with our feelings.

But God invites us to come to him with all of our feelings. And unlike a parent who is difficult to please, God welcomes us to be honest with him about what we're experiencing and feeling.

Gerry turned to God with all of her feelings after she was diagnosed.

I felt like a little child, nestling in God's bosom or sitting on his lap and saying, "I'm so scared. Help me!" It's pretty basic. I wanted so much to be a very spiritual person going through this, and I don't know what that's like. I don't know how we *are* spiritual, going through it; there's no code for that. All I could do was be real.

Gerry took her feelings to God with the trust and honesty of a child, which is what God invites us to do. The kingdom of heaven, Jesus said, is made up of people whose hearts are like those of little children (Mt 19:14).

Three of the feelings that we commonly face following a diagnosis of breast cancer are fear, anxiety and sadness. When we identify those feelings and take them to God, he promises to respond to us with the compassion and comfort that we need.

### Facing Our Feelings

Our emotional state immediately following our diagnosis may be one of numbness and disbelief. We're so overwhelmed with potential feelings that we may unconsciously shove them aside, so that we don't know *what* we're feeling. We perhaps tell ourselves that the diagnosis isn't real, that it didn't happen, that it *couldn't* happen to us. Everything within us shouts "No!"

Sherin, a single mother, didn't talk with anyone about her feelings after she was diagnosed with breast cancer. Aside from the fear that she wouldn't live to see her younger son graduate from high school, she wasn't sure what she was feeling.

> I felt I was walking around in another dimension. It was like knowing a deep, dark secret that I couldn't tell because I couldn't put it into words and no one would understand what I was feeling. I had this secret that I couldn't wipe from my mind, and I couldn't go back, and that depressed me. I didn't think I was depressed at the time, but I was carrying my feelings inside, and I gained weight and didn't care a lot about how I looked. I functioned every day without anyone knowing how I felt. Even though I had "let go and let God," I still had to accept the fact that my life had changed and that it would never be the same.

Although we might fool our conscious minds for a while, our bodies are never fooled. They soon begin to show signs of stress. Gerry found that she often couldn't finish a sentence. She would stop in the middle and then ask, "What's *wrong* with me?" And Connie lost twelve pounds in about ten days, because she didn't feel like eating.

When we begin to accept the reality of the diagnosis, our feelings can come crashing down on us. Feelings such as fear, anxiety and sadness. And maybe anger or disappointment or a sense of guilt. But we may not want to acknowledge such feelings to God or to others. A widespread belief among Christians is that the only emotions that are acceptable to God are the positive ones. If we're afraid, we're not following the Scriptures that say, "Do not fear"; if we allow ourselves to feel anger, it has to be "righteous anger"; if we're sad or depressed, we're not allowing the "joy of the Lord" to fill our hearts; if we're anxious, we're disobeying the command to "not be anxious about anything."

Some of us have no problem accepting so-called negative emotions. We might believe that all emotions are a gift from God, and so we have learned to be honest with him and with close friends about all that we're feeling. We might think of the Psalms, in which David felt free to cry out to God with such painful questions as "Why, O LORD, do you reject me and hide your face from me?" (Ps 88:14).

But when our lives are suddenly threatened by breast cancer, we may find it difficult to face the depths of our emotions, and we may not see them as a gift. We know we can't make the fear, anxiety, sadness and other unpleasant feelings go away simply by praying more or trying harder or claiming a Scripture. And yet we need to know that God accepts us in the midst of what we're feeling.

Our feelings about our diagnosis are probably mixed. Fear may be the predominant feeling. Anxiety and sadness may be tied for second place one evening, and by the next morning one or the other may have displaced the fear. Somewhere inside us may lurk some anger, disappointment or guilt feelings. Our mixed feelings can fluctuate from hour to hour. We need God to help us identify what we're feeling and help us respond to those feelings.

### Facing Our Fears

Chief among our fears is that we're going to die and that it may be soon and it may be painful. Because we all know people who have died of cancer, we tend to associate cancer with death. So the moment *we're* diagnosed with cancer, we wonder if we're next. Margaret, for example, describes the fear of dying that she used to experience: "It's that initial response that stops everything cold; it goes into suspended animation, and life just stops." Gerry wondered, after hearing her diagnosis, if she should plan her memorial service. And Connie, who was told she had a virulent form of cancer, was concerned about having time to "get things in order. I know I'm going to go to heaven," she says. "But wondering how I was going to get there made me fearful, because of the pain and the unknown."

No matter what we believe about life after death, we tend to fear death itself—or specifically the process of dying. We're afraid of how the intense, ongoing pain might feel when our bodies break down and quit functioning. We're afraid of being confined to a bed and having to depend on others to take care of our every need. We're afraid of having to say good-bye to those we love. Our fear of dying is useful in one way: it motivates us to do everything possible to survive. But it's also an all-consuming power that only God can help us face. We need him to walk through that fear with us.

It's almost impossible to ask ourselves *Am I going to die?* without also asking *What will happen to my family?* Margo's biggest fear when she was diagnosed was that her children would be left to grow up without their mother. That's not an unusual fear among mothers, but Margo had already seen what it could be like. Her husband, Wally, had lost his first wife in an automobile accident when his children were young, and Margo had helped Wally raise them through adolescence and into adulthood. Remembering how they had been impacted by their mother's death, she was frightened that the two children born to her and Wally may have to suffer the same loss.

> Our kids were the same ages as two of Wally's kids when their mother died, and I thought, *This is unbelievable*—the idea of the kids not having a mom; I couldn't deal with it. I knew that Wally would suffer, but the kids—. The pain for *them* would be indescribable. The loss, the abandonment, the emptiness, the absence of a role model and the ages of those kids—that's what my fear was. It's not right; it's not fair; it's horrible to lose a mom. How could this happen to me, not once, but twice?

While it's difficult for us to think of all that we would lose— particularly our close relationships—if we died, it's even more difficult to think of what our young children would have to endure in losing their mother. But we may also have deep fears about what our older children, our husbands and other family members would have to endure.

Our fear about what would happen to our families is just as real as our fear about dying. And we have a God who wants to help us with all of our fears.

### Facing Our Anxiety

We may become anxious after our diagnosis because we suddenly have no idea what will happen next week or next month or next year. Questions constantly swarm around our minds like mosquitos at a warm riverbank. *Will I have to lose a breast? If I need chemotherapy, will I lose my hair and feel sick all the time? How will I look? Will my husband still find me attractive? How many of my normal activities will I have to give up, and for how long? Will my family be OK while I'm trying to get well?* And perhaps most important, *Will my treatments save my life?* Suddenly our normal lives screech to a halt and dreams are put on hold while our minds spin in a frenzy of uncertainties.

Viola, who has had several recurrences of breast cancer, remembers how she responded the first time she was diagnosed.

> I cried with the doctor when I found out I probably had cancer. Then I went to a phone booth and called my friend Diane. I cried with her, and she prayed with me over the phone. My mind was racing from *Am I going to live?* to *I've got to get the laundry done, groceries bought,* and so on, *before I go to the hospital.*

Viola felt ill-equipped to face all the uncertainties that loomed in her future. But acknowledging her anxieties to a friend helped Viola to acknowledge her anxieties to God as well. And soon her anxieties diminished.

Our anxieties about having breast cancer may so overwhelm us that we can barely function. Maybe we can't even pray. When that happens, if we can acknowledge our anxieties to a friend who is willing to pray for us, we can be greatly helped. God understands those times, and he's ready to comfort us.

## Facing Our Sadness

Sadness settles into our hearts when we've begun to accept the reality of our breast cancer. We may experience deep sorrow over all the ways that our lives—and our perspectives—may change as the result of our diagnosis.

As with any major crisis, the experience of breast cancer can make us more acutely aware of how little control we have over our lives and how much we need God. We know that life is short and that horrible things can happen to good people. But whether that knowledge is a sudden revelation resulting from our diagnosis or a reminder of what we've long understood, we grieve over the possible loss of our dreams and hopes for the future.

Rachel grieved over those possible losses, including a loss of innocence about the future:

> I had always thought, *I'll live to be ninety-five years old; I have all these long-lived people in my family.* I think I was a pretty practical person, but I loved to dream about the future and think about the future as wonderful. Well, all of a sudden, at age forty-five, I'm brought up short, and I'm thinking, *Will I be around next Christmas?* Those are hard things to think about when you've been a person who's lived life pretty much in a fun way—in lightheartedness, in those little-girl feelings. I realized that I couldn't live that way, knowing that I was now living with something that made me vulnerable and that would always be there. I knew that my life was forever changed—that it would never, ever be the same again.

After Bonita was diagnosed, she experienced a deep sadness that turned into depression. In fact, she became too depressed to take proper care of herself. When her husband left for work each morning—on the days that he couldn't work at home—he drove Bonita to her parents' house so that she wouldn't be alone. "I was basically eating and sleeping," Bonita says, "and trying to smile for my children and trying not to let them see me sad, because they were young. But that was all I could really do."

God understands our sadness about having breast cancer. The Psalms are full of expressions of sadness: "How long must I wrestle with my thoughts and every day have sorrow in my heart?" (Ps 13:2); "My soul is weary with sorrow" (Ps 119:28); and "My eyes grow weak with sorrow, my soul and my body with grief" (Ps 31:9). When we acknowledge our sadness to God, we invite him to comfort us.

### Expressing Our Feelings to God

Margaret's face went hot, and her hands and feet were tingling. The doctor's verdict was sending shock waves through her body. On the way to her appointment, she had tried to imagine the worst, based on the tests she had undergone and the back pain she was experiencing. *Gall bladder surgery*, she had hypothesized. She hated having surgery, so she had asked God to prepare her for the news.

But it wasn't her gall bladder. The breast cancer that supposedly had been wiped out eight years earlier by chemotherapy was back, and it had spread to her liver and spine. Her doctor guessed she would survive no more than five months—maybe a bit longer with chemotherapy. "Help me, Jesus!" were the only words Margaret could utter. She had prayed the same prayer after her diagnosis eight years ago.

In the midst of Margaret's shock waves—about ten seconds after she heard the news from her doctor—she felt a peace and an acceptance of the diagnosis settle over her that she knew was from God. And she realized that he was answering both her simple cry for help and her earlier request that he prepare her for the diagnosis.

God knows what we need even before we ask him for it: "Before a word is on my tongue you know it completely, O LORD" (Ps 139:4). He didn't need Margaret to spell out the intricacies of her fears and needs before he would listen and respond. "Some of the words never came to my lips, because I was incapable of finding them," Margaret says. "It amazes me that when we are so inarticulate with God, he understands our needs anyway and goes ahead of us." Even when the best we can manage is a heavenward cry for help, we can be assured that God hears us.

Sometimes we don't turn to God because we're afraid of how he'll respond. It's ironic that although the first question on our minds after our diagnosis is usually *Am I going to die?* that question is one that many of us don't want to ask God. While the question looms like a dark cloud over our heads, we fight with all our power to make the answer become no. For

Margaret, it wasn't a question. She had just been told, implicitly, that she was going to die. And she turned to God with a general request for help. But she was able to do so because God was already responding to her fear of dying.

Margaret became unafraid of dying, she said, *after* she found out that she was going to die of breast cancer. And the peace that she received from God immediately after hearing the diagnosis has never stopped. She does sometimes fear the *process* of dying, however.

> Every time there's a fear, I have to ask God to come and help me with it. And I'm learning to remember that he is totally present, in his entire essence, not only indwelling me but right here with me. And that I don't have to be afraid, but he's going to go through this with me. I believe that with all my heart. He's going to be with me through the whole thing, and he's not going to allow me to go through anything that he knows I can't bear or that my husband can't bear.

By asking God to help her with her fear of the unknown each time she experiences it, Margaret finds that she regularly experiences God's peace in response to her request.

God offers us peace in response to our anxieties as well as to our fears. How many times have you heard someone—maybe yourself—say, "I know I'm not supposed to feel anxious, but . . . "? Many of us of us feel guilty when we hear or read the Scripture "Do not be anxious about anything" (Phil 4:6). We tend to assume that it's our responsibility to get rid of our anxiety, and until we do so, God is displeased with us. However, the remainder of that verse is an invitation: "but in everything, by prayer and petition, with thanksgiving, present your requests to God." We might reword the beginning of the verse to say, "Instead of trying to manage our anxiety by ourselves. . . . " God is urging us to bring all of our anxieties, all of our overwhelming fears and sorrows, to him. God cares about our anxious feelings because he cares for us (see 1 Pet 5:7). He may take our anxieties away, or he may help us endure them, but he promises to respond to us. And he does not reprimand us for feeling anxious.

One of the psalmists wrote, "I believed; therefore I said, 'I am greatly afflicted'" (Ps 116:10). The psalmist believed in a God who is good, merciful, loving, attentive, gracious, righteous, full of compassion, strong, faithful, responsive, and worthy of praise. Because he believed in this kind of God, he boldly cried out to God about his affliction, knowing that God would hear him and respond with compassion and love.

We also can boldly cry out to God, knowing that he wants to listen to our fears, anxieties, sadness—all of our feelings—about having breast cancer. We don't need to be afraid that he is displeased with our feelings or that he has better things to do than listen to us "complain." Because he is a good God who is deeply interested in each of us, we can say to him, "I am greatly afflicted"—by our fear that we'll die, by our anxieties about the unknown, by our sadness over how our lives will change or by any other feelings.

### Receiving Help from God

Elena was scheduled to have a CAT scan, and she was afraid. Her doctor suspected that she had cancer in her liver and in other areas besides her breast. A few days before the appointment, Elena visited a local church that her sister had recommended. After the worship service, Elena told one of the church leaders about her diagnosis and upcoming CAT scan, and he immediately gathered a small group of people to pray for her. The group's prayers had a significant effect on Elena.

> When we were praying, there was something so beautiful I felt. I felt that God was with me at that moment. I felt like a lot of energy came into my body. And I said, "They are not going to find cancer in my liver or under my arm or in my neck. Whatever they find, they're going to find it only in my breast."

What Elena believed that she was hearing from God turned out to be correct. The scan showed no cancer anywhere except in her breast. God had responded to Elena's fear even before she had the scan.

Margaret believes that the peace she experienced ten seconds after hearing her doctor's diagnosis was only the first of several gifts she received from God. Driving home alone from the doctor's office afterward, she was reminded of Romans 12:1: "Therefore, I urge you, brothers, in view of God's mercy, to offer your bodies as living sacrifices, holy and pleasing to God—this is your spiritual act of worship." Mar-

garet knew immediately what God was saying to her. "He wanted to do
something new in my life, and it was going to require that I give up
everything I have, including my life. And I agreed with him. Now, that's
a miracle."

God doesn't always give us immediate peace. Sometimes he allows
us to feel the depths of our fears, anxieties and sadness. And sometimes
he seems silent, in spite of our persistent pleas for his response. But he
does promise to respond. And we can expect, through his response, to
experience more of his presence.

Although Gerry reacted with shock when she found out that the
walnut-size lump she had discovered was malignant, her spiritual
reflexes pointed her in a helpful direction.

> I thought, *What do I do, and how do I come to grips with this?* But my next
> thought was, *I will go to the Rock.* So I was looking for psalms that spoke
> "rock language"—God's strength—and those were the psalms that com-
> forted me. I wanted something immutable and immovable. Something
> I could push against that would not give way. I wanted strong reminders
> of God's power and strength and protection.

Sometimes it helps to search the Scriptures—especially the Psalms,
which are rich with expressions of feeling—to find a passage that
specifically describes our sadness. Joan, along with Gerry, found the
Psalms helpful.

> When I found out that my bones were affected, I related to Psalm 34,
> which talks about the bones. Verse 20, "He protects all his bones, not
> one of them will be broken," was one that I was really hanging on to. I
> thought, *Well, maybe he might think of healing me yet.* That was a hard one,
> because I thought, *What does that really mean—"And none of them will be
> broken"*? But that psalm also says, "The LORD is close to the broken-
> hearted and saves those who are crushed in spirit" [v. 18] and "I will
> extol the LORD at all times; his praise will always be on my lips" [v. 1]. So
> I said, "Yes, Lord, I will praise you, no matter what."

Joan has had special prayer services on her behalf at various times,
and she has always featured that psalm as one of the Scripture readings,
because of its emphasis on praising God for his goodness no matter
what is happening to us.

The shock of being diagnosed with breast cancer might paralyze us so that we can't even pray Margaret's simple prayer, "Help me, Jesus." However, we needn't feel guilty. We're told that the Holy Spirit "helps us in our weakness" by praying for us, with "groans that words cannot express" (Rom 8:26). When we're unable to pray, we can also ask others to pray on our behalf. The apostle Paul says that we need to carry each other's burdens (Gal 6:2), and that includes allowing others to help us carry the burdens that are too heavy for us to carry alone. When our feelings are so deep that we can't pray, we can ask other people to do the praying for us. And when we're able at last to talk to God ourselves, we can feel free to express to him all of our fears, anxieties, sadness and other feelings.

We have a God who accepts us as we are and invites us to bring all our feelings and experiences to him. He understands our fear, anxiety and sadness: "The cords of death entangled me, the anguish of the grave came upon me; I was overcome by trouble and sorrow" (Ps 116:3; the *Good News Bible* translates the last phrase "I was filled with fear and anxiety"). And he promises to help us: "For I am the LORD, your God, who takes hold of your right hand and says to you, Do not fear; I will help you" (Is 41:13). Whenever we turn to God and tell him our feelings, we invite him to respond to us; we invite him to be toward us the same compassionate God that the writers of the Bible experienced. And God promises to respond to us with compassion.

---

**Here are some suggestions for responding to your fear, anxiety and sadness:**

■ Talk with some compassionate friends about your feelings, even if you don't want to. Doing so can cause the fear, anxiety and sadness to diminish.

■ If you can, share all your concerns with God. For some examples of prayers from the Bible, turn to the Psalms; the third psalm is a good place to start. Look also for verses in the Psalms that describe God with such words as *refuge, strength, hope, mercy* and *love*. Be alert to God's possible responses.

■ Find an oncologist that you feel you can trust—one who stays up-to-date on the latest treatments. Having good relationships with your doctors can lessen your fears and anxieties.

■ Avoid reading newspaper and magazine articles that include statistics on breast cancer survival rates. Remember that God has your life in his hands.

■ Educate yourself about your type of cancer. Go to a medical library, and ask the reference librarian for help.

■ Ask friends to pray for you and with you. If you find that you can't pray, be assured that God will respond to their prayers for you.

■ Do at least one thing each day that nurtures you: listen to music, read a good book, take a walk. Expect to receive some comfort from God through these activities.

# 3

# RESPONDING TO FEELINGS OF ANGER, DISAPPOINTMENT & GUILT

Gerry's fear that she would die of breast cancer gave way to anger when she was suddenly being told what to do and when and where to do it by doctors whom she had never met. Margo was "deeply disappointed" that God had allowed her to have breast cancer, because she held on to the subconscious belief that God rewards righteous living with health and long life. And Bonita struggled with guilt feelings when she realized that her faith in God wasn't conquering her anxiety about having breast cancer.

Experiencing feelings of anger, disappointment and guilt is normal when we've been diagnosed with breast cancer. We're angry that this insidious disease has invaded our bodies and is turning our lives upside down. We may be disappointed that God didn't protect us from it. And we may struggle with guilt feelings that we perhaps brought this disease upon ourselves, that we'll cause grief and inconvenience to others or that our faith seems weak. But the same God who invites us to come to him with our fear, anxiety and sadness invites us to bring our anger, disappointment and guilt feelings to him as well.

### Responding to Feelings of Anger

Gerry found it helpful to express her anger.

> Right after my diagnosis, my surgeon called me and said, "Now, I want you to do this," and he was using all these medical terms that I didn't know the meanings of, and I didn't know how to find out about them, and there was no acknowledgment that this might be a troubling time for me. I was furious with him. I didn't say that to him on the phone, but I wanted to just commit mayhem in my kitchen. I wanted to open all my cupboard doors and break all my dishes; I could very easily have gone berserk.
> Here I was, my life totally out of control. Too much of what I couldn't handle was delivered *bing-bing-bing,* like that, and then I was being steamrolled again. All these things, I'm sure, touched on very deep fear, and so there was a good deal of anger. Mostly, it was in the presence of my husband, and he gave me the entire arena. I would say, "I am so angry!" And he would say, "I know; I understand." Just having that anger affirmed let me be comfortable with being angry. And having expressed it, it would pass.

God gave us anger as an alarm system to tell us when something is not as he designed it, and breast cancer is certainly not part of his design. So our anger might help us by prompting us to ask questions, such as, "Why is God allowing this to happen?" "Why is this happening *now?*" or "Why me?" Although we may not get direct answers to those specific questions, asking them will likely sharpen our spiritual senses so that we can recognize the responses that God places in our path.

Ironically, many of us don't routinely turn to God with our anger. Here we are, God's dearly loved children who need the help of our loving Father, and we avoid talking with him about one of the most powerful phenomena of human experience. There are many possible reasons for this avoidance, but probably the most common one is our belief, conscious or unconscious, that anger is sin and until we confess our sin of anger to God there's no discussion.

The Bible does not condemn anger as sin, however. " 'In your anger do not sin': Do not let the sun go down while you are still angry," the apostle Paul writes (Eph 4:26), quoting David. This Scripture implies that anger itself is not a sin, but that we need to respond promptly and constructively to the *cause* of our anger. The alternative is either to respond to our anger destructively—for example, by raging at others or at ourselves—or to deny our anger, which is another way of responding destructively. When we deny our anger we separate ourselves from our true feelings and also from others and from God. Then our anger turns into bitterness. But we can choose instead to respond to our anger constructively by telling God or some other trustworthy person about our anger and explaining why we're angry.

God wants to help us with all our emotional struggles, including anger, and he gave us a model in Jesus, who expressed anger at least twice on earth (see Mk 3:5; Mt 21:12-13; Mk 11:15-17). In addition, the book of Hebrews tells us that God, who sees everything, will always be gracious to us when we come to him.

> For we do not have a high priest who is unable to sympathize with our weaknesses, but we have one who has been tempted in every way, just as we are—yet was without sin. Let us then approach the throne of grace with confidence, so that we may receive mercy and find grace to help us in our time of need. (Heb 4:15-16)

As our high priest who knows every angry feeling that we ever face, Jesus sympathizes with us. This is a concept that I have difficulty grasping. But whenever it makes some headway into my heart, I realize once again how much I want to talk with this God who sympathizes with my anger about having breast cancer. I want to ask him my "why" questions and receive his responses. We often don't understand our anger while we're feeling it in its raw state, but when we go to God, he will listen to us, help us to identify the specific causes of our anger, comfort us, share with us (sometimes) his purpose in what we're going through, direct us in what to do next and strengthen us to do it. He might respond to us through a passage in the Bible, or through a mental picture, or through images of nature, or through the words of a friend or family member (not only in person but sometimes in letters or phone calls), or through a sense of what he is saying or through a host of other sources. But he will respond.

These things don't all normally happen in just one conversation with God; that would overload us, and God promises not to give us more than we can receive. But we can expect to always "receive mercy and find grace" to help us in our times of anger.

## Responding to Feelings of Disappointment

Some of the women I interviewed said they felt overwhelmed about being diagnosed with a deadly disease when they had least expected it. As a result, some of them initially felt disappointed that God had not met their expectations.

*"Why me?"* Although we might ask ourselves "Why me?" after our diagnosis, we might find it difficult to ask God that question. Margo had no trouble taking that question to God, however. She describes her main reaction as "disappointment" that God had allowed her to have cancer.

> I was heartbroken. From my background and the teaching I'd received, it was clear in my mind that if you were good you would be rewarded—which, of course, is outrageous, and it's not good theology at all, but I did believe that at some level. I'd been a faithful, faithful follower of Jesus all my life. I never did the rebellion routine, and I never smoked and I never drank and I never—. I had a real "righteous" mentality. [*Laughing*] I'd been so righteous that certainly God saw me with favor. And this was a cruddy payoff. What does "clean living" give you, if you get this rotten disease and die? What good does it do to eat right and care about your body? It didn't make any sense to me, because I thought I had been faithful; therefore, I would be rewarded with a long and fruitful life, and I would be exempt from deep sorrow. And, you know, I used to sing with my brother, "God hath not promised skies always blue, Flower strewn pathways all our lives thro'; . . . But God hath promised strength for the day."[1] So I knew in my head that it wasn't that life would be great but that God would be *with* me. But there was also some "If you're really good, God rewards you" stuff going on in my head.
>
> And because I'd gotten cancer when I never thought I would, I couldn't *predict* anything. I just didn't have any framework now to make *any* decisions about life. So, Why me? was a huge question on my mind.

Of the many Christian women I've talked with who have experienced breast cancer, I've found very few who say they have asked, "Why me?" Some women don't ask that question because they see it as a way of accusing God of cruelly targeting them for evil. Others don't ask it because they would expect God to respond with something like, "Well, why *not* you?" Still others did ask God that question during earlier crises in their lives but have found God's peace in the midst of breast cancer and no longer feel the need to ask. Yet some women, like Margo, have asked why—not necessarily out of anger, but out of confusion and disappointment and a yearning for God to show them his purposes in their suffering.

As Margo struggled with some of her subconscious beliefs about God, she quickly realized that it was her church background, not the Bible, that had taught her wrongly. She had been implicitly trained in an ethic that God's good gifts are the rewards for hard work and faithfulness, but her breast cancer experience gave her a greater awareness of how little control she has over her own life. Breast cancer had "threatened my theology," she says. "But it needed to."

All of us need at times to have our theology threatened. And that is sometimes what happens when we ask God, "Why me?" When our defenses are uncovered and we ask God why he's allowing us to have breast cancer, we can begin to see more clearly what we truly believe about him. God then gives us the opportunity to reject any wrong assumptions and embrace the truth: that he loves us individually, that he is full of grace and mercy toward us, and that he is always with us to help us endure any threat to our lives as well as any threat to our theology. Whether he reminds us through Scripture of his loving presence, or he brings us gifts of love and compassion through others, or he gives us a sense of purpose in what we're experiencing or he supernaturally puts our hearts at rest, we can be confident that he will respond when we ask, "Why me?"

*"Haven't I had enough?"* Sherin had been physically abused for nearly her entire thirteen-year marriage and had undergone seven surgeries, most of them major. When she was diagnosed with breast cancer, she could not understand why God was taking away the contentment and peace that she had finally found only a short time before.

When Judy was diagnosed with breast cancer, she was already battling two chronic illnesses. In addition, she had recently undergone a hysterectomy, had even more recently been hospitalized a third time for clinical depression and had found out that her mother's lymphoma had recurred and spread. Judy wondered how much more she could take.

Sarah had struggled since young adulthood with the disappointment that she would never be able to bear children. And she and her husband had faced obstacle after obstacle before they were finally able to adopt their two sons. So Sarah confesses to moments of feeling bitter that she must now fight breast cancer.

And Viola, who has endured several recurrences of breast cancer, has had times of wondering if there was another Viola someplace who was supposed to get some of what she herself has gone through, "because *this* Viola can only handle so much."

We all know that bad things happen to good people. Bad things happen also to those who are already ill, injured, bereaved, anxious, discouraged, stressed, depressed and oppressed. Knowing that reality, however, does not keep us from feeling that God surely could make an exception in our case. And so Sherin, Judy, Sarah and Viola, along with others of us, have asked God a common variation of the "why" question: "Haven't I had enough?"

When Sherin asked God that question she couldn't see any purpose for what she was experiencing. But God responded to her in a way she hadn't expected.

> When I trusted God for the healing of my body and mind, that was a test of my faith. I learned not to care what a situation looks like. It's not over until God says it's over. To encourage another heart, or even understand what they are going through, one would have had to go through a few trials to build strength and faith in the Lord. My faith has gotten stronger.

God responded to Judy by leading her to the Scripture verse that says, "Cast all your anxiety on him because he cares for you" (1 Pet 5:7). His answer to How much more can I handle? was that he would do the handling. "My responsibility," she says, "was to give my burdens to him."

Sarah found that God responded to her question by helping her to be more hopeful. She felt that he often told her not to be anxious and that he helped her to face breast cancer in ways that deepened her relationship with him.

Although Viola felt that her recurrences were stretching the limits of God's promise that he will never allow us to carry more than we're capable of carrying (1 Cor 10:13), her questions for God were full of faith.

> Each time I've had a recurrence, my first response has been, "I don't understand why I have to deal with this again. Was there something I was supposed to learn last time that I didn't? If I have to deal with this again, then there must be something you want me to do with it. Please make the open doors obvious."

When we ask God, "How much more can I handle?" what we really mean is "Can we stop now? I don't believe I can handle any more." God knows our emotional needs that prompt that question. He responds by assuring us of his care for us and by building our strength, our faith and our hope.

### Responding to Feelings of Guilt

It's normal to have guilt feelings even when we're not truly guilty. It's also normal to wonder if we've done something wrong. The onset of breast cancer can result in a barrage of guilt feelings that raise one or more questions in our minds: *Did I do something to cause my cancer?* or *Is my faith too weak?* We might also struggle with guilt feelings that we could possibly die and leave our children without a mother. Or guilt feelings that we might not die, whereas someone we care about did die of cancer.

*"Did I do something to cause my cancer?"* As creatures of control, we sometimes think that when something bad happens to us, we should have been able to prevent it. Our conscious, logical minds may rush to our defense: *Don't blame yourself; this was beyond your control.* But we can't help but wonder if we did something to cause our cancer, especially because of the popular emphasis on nutrition, exercise and other things we can do to reduce our risk. We might feel guilty that we didn't

take care of our bodies well enough to protect ourselves.

Once I got past the initial disbelief that I had breast cancer, I was assaulted with the questions What caused my cancer? and Is there something I could have done to prevent it? So I often talked with God about these mysteries. I didn't want to hear that I could have prevented my cancer, but I believed that God would either answer my questions or make me content not to know the answers.

I soon sensed that God wanted me to be concerned with what he was going to do through my experience with breast cancer rather than with what had caused it. I never felt it was wrong to ask him about it, though; asking had prepared my heart to receive God's response. And God's response was full of comfort and encouragement.

If stress can cause breast cancer, I figure that we increase our risk for recurrences simply by trying to determine how we got breast cancer. Jane, a college dean and mother who was diagnosed with breast cancer in 1993, struggled for a while with guilt feelings, because she wondered if she had stretched herself too far. "I put a lot of pressure on myself in terms of the kind of mother I want to be, the kind of dean I want to be," she says, "and that was my question: Did I do this by choosing to work?" Jane considers herself a traditional mother in many ways. One day when I talked with her, she had baked snickerdoodles at 6:30 that morning for an activity at her daughter's school before leaving home for a full day's work. "When the school needs baked goods, I'm always one to volunteer, and I just can't imagine buying them," she says. In addition, she enjoys cross-stitching and other handcrafts, which she tries to sandwich between spending time with her family and maintaining a full-time career. Knowing that she was often stressed by trying to serve both her family and the college, Jane fought momentary feelings of guilt that her breast cancer might have resulted from her choice to have a career.

Whenever the guilt feelings arose, however, Jane reminded herself that throughout her career she had asked God to show her if she should resign and devote all her time to her family. And continually she had had the sense—partly by observing her children and paying attention to their emotional needs—that God did not want her to stay at home. "The children are wonderful; people are amazed," she says. "And I think that God has honored that prayer and has cared for them." She found that God always alleviated her guilt feelings and gave her peace that her choice to have both a career and a family had not contributed to her cancer.

Joan, unlike Jane, had no guilt feelings the first time she was diagnosed with breast cancer. But when she had a recurrence, two people "spoke" to her about diet, and another person waved a giant bottle of vitamin C in her face and said, "Here. Take this." Joan then began thinking, *Did I do something wrong? Should I have eaten better?*

Joan discovered, as she sought answers to her questions, that God didn't seem nearly as concerned about what had caused her cancer as she was. However, she's glad that she tried to get some answers. "I want to know that I have done everything possible that I can do," she says. "And that was good for me to know, because I've come to more of an awareness that God is the one who's in control."

Rachel wondered what had caused her cancer, especially when she was diagnosed with colon cancer thirteen years after being treated for breast cancer. "I didn't drink, I didn't smoke, I ate everything in moderation, and I led a reasonably sensible life," she says. "I had been such a middle-of-the-road person that I was *dull*." But in her quest for answers, God led her to some peaceful conclusions.

> I believe that God gives only good gifts and that I got cancer because I'm human. And part of our human dilemma is disease and illness. I had one relative who was just agonizing over the possible causes of cancer and trying to get all of her questions answered at my expense. I finally said, "You know, this isn't helpful to me at all. The greatest minds in the world don't know why, and *you and I* are expending energy on this question?" And I just let go of that.

We're wise to take good care of our bodies by doing a breast self-exam each month, getting regular professional health exams and mammograms, eating foods that are low in fat and high in fiber, exercising regularly, minimizing stress as much as possible, avoiding tobacco and drinking only a moderate amount of alcohol. But there's only so much we can do to merely reduce our risk of breast cancer; no one knows yet how to prevent it. If we struggle with guilt feelings because of our diagnosis, we can tell God about them and look for his responses. Only he can take away our guilt feelings and give us peace.

"*Is my faith too weak?*" From the time that Bonita was first diagnosed with breast cancer, she felt that she never trusted God enough. Her standard was the Scripture "Do not be anxious about anything" (Phil 4:6), which she found impossible to obey, because "I'm anxious about *everything,*" she says. So on top of struggling with anxiety, she struggled also with guilt feelings *about* her anxiety.

Although Bonita completed her breast cancer treatments in 1990, her struggles emerged again, in 1997, when she found another lump in her breast. The lump turned out to be benign, but until it was diagnosed she felt guilty once again about being anxious rather than having faith in God. Her wise father counseled her, "Bonita, you're human. And what you're feeling is OK. Trust in the Lord." She has seen progress recently in her ability to trust God and not feel guilty about her anxiety, and she now accepts the fact that she has strong moments and weak moments.

Bonita is not alone in feeling guilty about her faith. Many of us who have had breast cancer, or any other major crisis, have struggled with the same issue. But the struggle has resulted, for Bonita and for many others, in a stronger faith.

The Bible speaks often of God using the crises in our lives to strengthen our faith. We're told that the "testing" of our faith develops perseverance, and "perseverance must finish its work so that you may be mature and complete, not lacking anything" (Jas 1:3-4). I like to think of *testing* in this sense in the same way that a few of my schoolteachers used to introduce a written test with those altruistic words that I never trusted: "I hope you will learn something as you take this test." I used to bristle also at the verses in the Bible that talk about testing, until I realized that God, unlike my schoolteachers, does not need to test us so that he can find out how we're doing. He already knows. Rather, he tests us to show *us* how we're doing. Perhaps more important, his tests are opportunities for us to grow in our faith and to be encouraged by our growth. Like Job, who asked God questions and was commended for his perseverance (Jas 5:11), we can become stronger in our faith in the midst of having breast cancer.

God's compassion and mercy help us to persevere, no matter how weak our faith may seem. We feel anxious because we're human. But God understands our anxiety—and our guilt feelings *about* our anxiety. As we give those feelings to him, he strengthens our faith.

*Responding to other feelings of false guilt.* Feelings of false guilt can arise for many other reasons when we're experiencing breast cancer. And sometimes they arise within our family members. Margaret's mother had had breast cancer, and when Margaret was first diagnosed five years later, her mother felt guilty, as though she had passed the cancer on to Margaret genetically. "We had to do some long talks about how God is still in control," Margaret says, "and the fact that I don't blame her; there's no issue of blame at all."

Another possible source of false guilt is the fear of dying, and abandoning those who love us and need us. When Sherin, at age forty-three, discovered a lump in her breast, her first thought was, *How am I going to tell my children and my mother that I may not live?* She felt guilty, as if she were doing something to hurt them. "I was concerned about my mother's health if she found out," Sherin says. "And the guilt I felt was that I might die and leave my children without a mother. I was their only parent, and they needed me."

Viola, like Sherin, felt guilty because of how her cancer might affect those close to her. Viola's family and friends have had to watch her endure several recurrences of breast cancer. She tried several times to call off her dating relationship with Perry, whom she later married. He had lost his first wife to breast cancer, and Viola didn't think it was fair for him to have to risk repeating the experience. But he told her, "I'm old enough to know what's fair and what isn't, and I want to have as much time with you as I can."

Guilt feelings about possibly dying are commonly experienced by women who have breast cancer. But almost as common are guilt feelings about surviving. Judy, a children's librarian who was diagnosed with breast cancer, tells of a coworker who was diagnosed with inoperable cancer at the same time. As Judy listened to a counselor from their employee assistance program talk at a staff meeting soon after the coworker's diagnosis, she felt overcome with guilt that her own cancer was treatable and her coworker's cancer was not. When the coworker died about two months later, Judy continued to feel guilty.

I remember having some subtle, fleeting guilt feelings following my own diagnosis—guilt feelings about possibly dying *and* possibly surviving. I knew that the news of my diagnosis would upset my parents terribly. And it did. So I felt guilty about that, as if I had done something to hurt them. I was stunned to realize that what I was telling the people I loved had the power to shatter their sense of well-being, and I think that the cause-and-effect relationship led to feelings of false guilt. I felt guilty also that I would probably survive, when my friend Karen had died of breast cancer. It didn't make any sense that she should die, leaving her two-year-old daughter motherless, and I should go on living, even though I had no children and I was needed, so it seemed, by fewer people. I knew that my breast cancer was beyond my control and that blaming myself was absurd. But the guilt feelings were real.

I had several choices. I could ignore my feelings, hoping they would eventually go away. Or I could try to talk myself out of them by arguing, *It's not my fault that my parents are distressed about my diagnosis. There's nothing to feel guilty about.* Or I could take my guilt feelings to him who is called Wonderful Counselor (Is 9:6).

I'd like to say I chose wisely and that I immediately ran to God with my confusion. But I didn't. I vaguely remember instead doing all three things at separate moments—although the third was reduced to a faint heavenward cry for help. However, God responded to my cry anyway, by freeing me from guilt feelings. If I ever face a life-threatening crisis again—and I probably will—I hope that I would pray, "Search me, O God, and know my heart; test me and know my anxious thoughts. See if there is any offensive way in me, and lead me in the way everlasting" (Ps 139:23-24). When we tell God about our guilt feelings, we are inviting him to respond to us in a personal way—a way that comforts us with his peace.

A popular myth is that we have much more control over our own lives than we actually have. So when we're diagnosed with breast cancer, it's natural to feel guilty that we didn't do everything possible to prevent it. We might feel the urgency to pursue some possible answers, but no matter what we think we should have done differently, we can remind ourselves that our God is full of compassion and mercy and that, if we turn to him, he will lead us in "the way everlasting."

# 4

---

# RECEIVING
# HELP FROM
# OTHERS

O ne of the good things that may happen after our diagnosis is that we become surrounded by caring people who are eager to comfort and encourage us. They help us by listening attentively and then responding with kind words, hugs, practical help, prayer and other gifts. Because the Bible tells us that all good gifts come from God (Jas 1:17), we have an opportunity to recognize in each good gift that comes to us, and in each giver of the gift, the love of God toward us. And we can experience more of the goodness of God when we are willing to receive help from others.

### Learning to Receive

As Christians, and especially as Christian women, we tend to be self-sufficient givers, uncomfortable perhaps with other people doing things for us that we would normally do ourselves. We've been taught that it's better to give than to receive, that we must think of others first and ourselves last, that we must be models of selflessness, hospitality and generosity. Having absorbed the concept of giving into every molecule of our being, we volunteer for important tasks at church, drop what we're doing to listen to a friend's distress, and lay aside our own needs to help a total stranger. While such actions are admirable and are supported by the Bible, we hear their virtues emphasized so much that we tend to ignore the equally biblical concept of receiving good gifts.

But God tells us to ask him for whatever we need, because he is a generous Father who enjoys giving good gifts to his children (Mt 7:7-8, 11). And he often uses other people to provide what we've asked him for. How easily we forget that Paul's mandate to carry each other's burdens (Gal 6:2) includes allowing others to carry *our* burdens.

For some of us, our discomfort with having other people serve us might be rooted in how we define our self-worth. When Margaret was undergoing chemotherapy in 1989 she sometimes asked God, "Of what value am I when I'm so helpless?" As a successful bed-and-breakfast innkeeper, she had taken pride in anticipating the needs of others, making them feel welcome, providing them with comfortable lodgings and delighting their eyes, ears and taste buds. But her treatments made her so sick that she no longer could serve her guests, or anyone else, in tangible ways. For the first time in her life, Margaret struggled to find her self-worth.

She remembers on one winter day looking out the window of the inn that she and her husband owned on the Oregon coast. What she saw surprised her: a friend from church was in Margaret's garden, pulling weeds.

> I was overcome with a sense of helplessness and shame, that this dear person was serving me, rather than my serving her. I had always been the one that served; that's where I got my brownie points, and that's what being a bed-and-breakfast innkeeper for me was all about. As a child, I'd been taught that you serve others; that's where your value is. So when I was not able to serve and others were serving *me,* it was terribly upsetting.
>
> Finally, a friend got tough with me and said, "Did it occur to you that we might *need* to serve you but you're robbing us of an opportunity of service by insisting on doing it yourself?" That was what I needed to hear, of course.

Having questioned God about her value, Margaret began to recognize his answer: that her value is not based on her service to others.

Whatever the cause of our discomfort in receiving help might be, sometimes the best gift we can give to others is to allow them to help us. In doing so, we might be giving ourselves the even greater gift of experiencing God through the helpful acts of others. Besides, we may not have a choice. Overwhelmed with feelings (or else with shock) about our cancer and with the need to make treatment decisions, we may find it hard to function on some days. We need others to listen to us vent, pick up the kids, prepare dinner for our families or help us think straight.

But we do not become magically transformed from self-sacrificing givers into glad recipients overnight. If we're accustomed to always responding to the needs of others first, how do we suddenly change our thinking so that we can learn to receive from others?

There are a few things we can do to learn to receive. First, we need to *be patient with ourselves.* Any deliberate change in human behavior takes time, especially when we're overwhelmed by feelings.

Second, we need to *recognize and accept our present limitations.* We may be able to function at near-normal capacity, or we may need to hang a "Temporarily closed for repairs" sign on our souls as a notice to others and as a reminder to ourselves. Bonita, who was "basically not functioning" after her diagnosis, was glad when family members volunteered to go with her to doctor appointments.

> Once they said I had cancer—hey, there was no information you could have given me that I would have been able to remember. Sometimes I would click into the emotional aspects, and I wouldn't hear all the facts. And whoever went with me—my husband or my mom—would write down any kind of instructions, any kind of information. If something was not clear, they would ask for clarification. That was very helpful, because when I came home and I would wonder about something, they could even pull the paper out and say, "This is what the doctor said." It's important that somebody fills that role.

A third step in learning to receive is to *decide who we can express our needs to, and then do it.* We can start to rely on family members, certain friends and perhaps a few other cancer survivors to listen to us when we feel afraid or frustrated or angry about our cancer. We may or may not need to tell them, "I need you to listen sometimes to what I'm feeling." We might also ask family members to take on additional household chores, ask our coworkers to cover for us or suggest that our boss hire a temporary replacement, or ask friends and fellow church members to visit us, pray for us and be on call to occasionally help with meals, transportation, errands, babysitting and gardening.

Suppose, however, that we feel strong and healthy. Shouldn't we stick to our normal routines for as long as possible, so that we can feel normal? Perhaps. But we need to remember that our lives have been turned upside down. We have many decisions to make and feelings to respond to. Our families' lives have been turned upside down as well, and the feelings and changes that they experience—no matter how well they seem to be coping—will continually impact us. All of our decisions, all of the adjustments we need to make, take time. We cannot expect to stay in our normal routines and give adequate time to the important emotional, as well as practical, tasks that we now face. We therefore need to rely on others for help.

Our God is a God of help. And he uses people as his hands and feet and heart. When we're concentrating on getting well, we can express our needs to those who might be able to meet them. We need others to listen to us attentively, accept the feelings we express, hug us, pray for us, reassure us of their love and give us a hand with our daily chores. When we receive that kind of help, we are receiving gifts—gifts from those who help us and gifts through them from God.

### Recognizing Varieties of Help

Frieda received a gift of encouragement from God when she found a potted plant left on her doorstep by thoughtful friends. The card accompanying the plant said, "We're thinking of you; we know you're in God's hands, and we're praying that his strength will be yours"—or words to that effect. "Right then I *knew* that God was with me," she says. "I knew that, whatever happened, he held me firmly in his hand."

Assuming that the friends who had brought the plant had heard about her diagnosis, Frieda called them and discovered that they knew only that she had recently undergone a breast biopsy. They didn't know the outcome, much less that Frieda had heard the outcome that day. So Frieda was amazed that God had moved these friends to convey an important message to her at the time she most needed it.

Gifts of help from others can express compassion, encouragement, hope, confidence, faith and the reassurance that we're loved. A brief note from some friends gave me all of those gifts when it arrived one day in our mailbox, soon after John and I had sent out our Christmas letters in which we reported my recent short-lived experience with cancer. "Barbara, we were jolted to hear of your cancer," the husband wrote.

*Jolted.* Although it's not thought of as a comforting word, I felt comforted by it somehow. Then I realized why: it let me know that those friends felt what *I* had felt. I was comforted by their assurance that I was not alone in feeling jolted.

One of our greatest needs when we have breast cancer is for others to understand, even slightly, what we're feeling. And to be understood means that they listen to us. We don't want to hear stories about people who have survived breast cancer, nor assumptions about what we're feeling, nor judgments about what we say, nor any advice, particularly about the latest cancer "cures." We may not even want to hear Scripture verses. We need others to simply let us express our fears, our sadness or our anger about having cancer. And those who listen to us give us the most generous gift possible: the gift of themselves.

Perhaps we found it easy to accept help when we were first diagnosed. Friends may have overwhelmed us with kindness and compassion, and it felt good to be waited on for a change. But as long-term treatments wear on for weeks or months, we may become uncomfortable with all the attention. That has been Joan's experience. "People continued showering me with care," she says, "and I thought, *OK, now it's enough.* It's been ongoing for the last four years, and I think, *Don't you ever get sick of me?*" Yet Joan found that allowing others to help her enriched her relationships with them and reminded her that she was not alone.

Gerry had one more test to undergo—a bone scan—after completing five weeks of daily radiation treatments. Fatigued from the radiation and from the demanding schedule, and apprehensive about the procedure, she didn't want to go alone to get the scan, but her husband was out of town. So she called a friend and said, "I'm all out of 'brave.'

Can you go with me to take this test?" To Gerry's relief, the friend canceled a hair appointment and went with her.

The greatest help of all is not the meals and the babysitting and the transportation and the phone calls and other expressions of care that people give us—although those can be crucial. By far the greatest means of help is the reassurance that we're not alone. We need to know that others are with us, caring about us and trying to understand what we're experiencing. The most important element of a helpful act is not the act itself but our relationship with the person who performs it.

## Receiving Spiritual Help

After our diagnosis, it's important that we immediately find trustworthy spiritual support. For me, God had already provided that support before I knew I would need it. John and I were hiking with our friends Joe and Sally Ann on Mt. Tamalpais, just north of the Golden Gate Bridge, the day after I found out I had breast cancer. The plans had been made weeks in advance, and although I was still reeling from the shock of the diagnosis, there was no way I was going to miss that hike and the opportunity to be with friends.

Joe and Sally Ann didn't know yet about the news from my doctor. I had waited to tell them in person, but when we met them that morning I wasn't ready to disrupt our day. As the four of us trudged up the mountain, breathing the fresh, coastal air and relishing the crunch of leaves under our feet, I wondered when and how I could manage to speak the words "I have breast cancer and I will probably have to have a mastectomy" before my tears would make a mess of me.

At lunchtime we chose some flat-topped boulders for our picnic benches, and I decided to tell Joe and Sally Ann the news after we'd eaten but while we were still seated. I don't think I tasted my sandwich; I felt like I was swallowing sawdust. And I have no idea what words spilled out of my mouth after "Before we go, there's something I need to tell the two of you."

What I do remember is that the instant I quit talking, Joe and Sally Ann and John were at my side, with Sally Ann holding me as I sobbed uncontrollably. After a few minutes, they asked if they could pray for me. Although I soon forgot everything they prayed, I'll never forget the warmth of their hands on my shoulders and God's presence with me in the cool silence of the forest.

That was only the beginning of the continual prayer support that I received. About twenty people gathered around me to pray for me after church the next morning; several women friends came to my home twice, on my request, to pray for me and listen to God on my behalf; and I was amazed at the notes I received, not only from friends but also from the *mothers* of friends, saying that they were praying for me and that their Bible study groups or Sunday school classes were praying for me. I felt loved, and I knew from the depths of my soul that I was safe in God's hands.

God does not want us to face breast cancer alone. He is with us, and he sends us brothers and sisters who can pray for us and make us more aware of his presence with us. (For more information about finding spiritual support, see appendix A.)

### "If There's Anything I Can Do . . ."

If you have breast cancer, you have probably been told many times, "If there's anything I can do. . . . " You may have had a ready answer: "Thanks. I'll let you know." And then you did. Or perhaps you answered in the same gracious way, but you thought to yourself, *What does this person mean by "anything"?* and you decided never to impose on that person by asking for help.

Ironically, an open-ended offer of help ("anything, any time") can put pressure on us, the potential recipients. Some people make that kind of offer because they sincerely want to help us but they don't know how. Others, however, may figure that we won't take them up on their offer and they'll be off the hook; they can thereby appear gracious without going to any trouble. But as we try to discern who is sincere in the offer and who isn't, we begin to worry about offending someone by either ignoring an offer that's sincere or accepting one that's insincere. As a result, our burdens are made heavier rather than lighter.

Bonita and Nancy were quick to answer those who made open-ended offers of help and who believed that God answers prayer: "Pray for me." "For others," says Nancy, "I just said I'd let them know. And never did."

Perhaps a better solution to the dilemma—a solution that might get us the practical help that we need—is to respond with something like this:

> I'm going to need a *number* of people to help me with a variety of tasks—including transportation to the clinic every day, dinner five nights a week, housecleaning once a week and occasional child care. You don't need to give me an answer now, but if you'd like to consider doing one of those tasks occasionally and you can let me know next week, that would be great. If you realize, though, that you can't help, I'll understand.

This kind of response gives choices to the person who sincerely wants to help, and it gives the person who isn't ready to make a commitment the opportunity to back out of the offer without feeling embarrassed.

If you belong to a church or other organization that is willing to publicize the personal needs of its members in a bulletin or newsletter, consider making your list of needs known in that way. Once the word gets around, you'll likely receive more offers of specific help and fewer offers of "anything, any time." Best of all, your load will be lightened.

### Responding to "Help" That Isn't Helpful

Some people want to help us but don't know how. They feel awkward, or they're afraid of saying the wrong thing. And some of them do say the wrong thing. They may be people who care about us, and so they want to do something for us. But their attempts fall flat and make us feel worse. So how should we respond to these unhelpful but well-meaning people?

One woman I interviewed—we'll call her Cheryl for this example—had a particularly aggressive kind of cancer, but a friend of hers couldn't understand why Cheryl would consider chemotherapy or other forms of treatment that would involve side effects. "Why torture yourself?" she asked Cheryl. "Why don't you simply enjoy your quality of life for as long as you can?" *In other words,* thought Cheryl, *why not just give up and die?*

Having recently read a verse in the Bible that says "choose life" (Deut 30:19), Cheryl had already decided to "hit this cancer with everything that I possibly can and let the Lord do the rest." And so it hurt her to not be supported by her friend in what might be a life-or-death decision. Cheryl did not try to talk further with her friend about that issue, but she silently forgave her.

Choosing to not respond to the person who is being unhelpful might be the best decision occasionally, but at other times we may save ourselves from further anxiety by speaking up. Several women I talked with said that a few friends and family members were unhelpful to them by saying, "Call and let me know how you're doing." These women responded, "I won't have the energy to make phone calls, but you're welcome to call *me*." They added that they often weren't able to talk on the phone but that family members had volunteered to give callers a medical update.

Some people try to help us by giving us overwhelming amounts of medical information. Margo remembers someone sending her a book that discussed the details of chemotherapy. "I read about five pages, closed it up and said, 'Who needs *this?*'" And then she threw the book away. Margo did later undergo chemotherapy, but what she needed first was emotional support, not impersonal efforts to educate her about possible treatments.

Sometimes it's simpler to avoid people who tend to be unhelpful, especially those who are not actively involved in our lives. "I didn't need to have my condition trivialized, and I felt in some instances it was," says Gerry, who distanced herself from a few people. "I didn't have time to think about other people's discomfort with what I was going through. They could work that out themselves."

If we value our relationships with those who are unhelpful to us, we might want to risk honestly telling them when their attempts to help us are hurting us. Although they might respond defensively, there's a chance that they will regret hurting us and tell us so, and they may try to become more understanding. When they respond that way, our mutual relationships can become closer and stronger.

### Telling Health Care Professionals What We Need
We need to feel that the professionalism of our doctors and other members of our health care team goes beyond helping us survive; we

need to feel that they want to help us survive because they care about us as individuals. When these needs are not being met, we may find it helpful to speak out. Gerry surprised herself one day by speaking out to a doctor she was seeing for the first time:

> He came into the examining room holding a file folder instead of having his hand out to greet me. I knew he was using the file folder to shield himself from me, and I thought, *Oh, my! I'm in trouble now.* Usually, you expect the doctor to walk into the room and say, "Hi! I'm Dr. Jones!" and you know you're probably in good company. But this doctor began with, "Well, we'll look at this file and have an examination, and then we'll get acquainted." But I threw up my arms and said, "Oh, no! *No!* First we'll get acquainted, and *then* we'll talk about the other."
>
> I think it shook him. I had just blurted it out. Since then, I've come to love that doctor, but in that first visit I felt so utterly vulnerable. I wanted the medical people, in particular, to respect me as a person and to know that there are emotions attached to this breast. A lot of them.

It's difficult to bare our breasts to a stranger, even though that stranger is a doctor. So we need to feel comfortable with that doctor. Gerry's experience with her new doctor motivated her to speak out about a similar situation a few days later, when she went for a dress rehearsal of her radiation treatments.

> Everyone was in there, it seemed—the doctor, his assistant, the head technician, her assistant. There were four or five people around me, looking at a very intimate part of my body and talking about it as if I weren't even there. They were not paying a bit of attention to me; they did not speak my name; they did not say, "Good morning." They just told me to lie on this slab, and then they began taking a picture of me. And I was crying because of this indifference. I closed my eyes; I would not look at the camera. When I left, nobody even said good-bye, and I was furious. So when I went the next day, I told the chief technician, "I can't go through this all summer long. I don't want to be anonymous here, I don't want to be a number, and I don't want to be ignored. I want somebody to use my *name.*" It had been a humiliating experience, and I told her I felt like a piece of meat.
>
> She said, "Well, that was our fault, and we're doing something wrong here." She *heard* me. Telling her how I felt was hard, but I knew I had to speak up. I was a whole person going through this. It didn't have to do

with my breast only; it was *all* of me going through this. And I was determined to be *me*, no matter what. So I knew I couldn't go back there the next day unless I had some help and support.

The whole staff was lined up *the next day,* greeting me with, "Hi, Gerry! Hello, Gerry! How are *you,* Gerry?" It made us all laugh. And I felt like singing and dancing, going into the treatment room. I'd gotten their attention and cooperation. Hurray!

Now when I go back for checkups, they are obviously very glad to see me. It's a very affirming thing, when you can say to hospital staff or doctors, "Look, I need this. Can you help me?" and you are heard. I think I was forced to ask for things like that along the way—things that I needed in order to survive the treatment process. And I learned how to do that better.

The more medical professionals we see, the more likely we will encounter one or two who focus on our physical conditions with no thought for our feelings. However, if we tell them how their behavior is affecting us—with an emphasis on our feelings, so that our words don't sound like an accusation—they may be willing to change. Although the last thing we might feel inclined to do right now is to confront others about their unhelpful behavior, we may make our breast cancer experience much more bearable by doing so. And we may eventually find that some of the unhelpful people—including those in the medical establishment—have joined the ranks of the supportive friends in our lives.

---

**Here are a few guidelines for receiving help from others:**

■ Learn what you can about your type of cancer. Get a second and perhaps a third medical opinion. Medical professionals can be a gift from God. Ask them for help.

■ Find out who in your church and among your friends and neighbors has had breast cancer. Don't look to them for medical advice, but ask them what particularly helped them in their experiences with cancer.

■ Ask as many friends as possible to pray for you daily.

■ Take an adult family member or close friend with you to doctor appointments. Ask that person to write down any instructions or new information given by the doctor.

■ Try to decide ahead of time what you might want to say, if anything, to people who will respond to you in unhelpful ways.

---

# 5

---

# SEEKING GOD'S WISDOM ABOUT TREATMENT

WhHen we've been traumatized by the news that we have cancer, we're not in the best place emotionally to decide what kind of treatment has the best shot at saving our lives. But we know that not to decide would be the worst thing we could do. We might turn to our doctors, with a sense of helplessness, and say, "Tell me what to do." Or we might get to know our local reference librarians, become familiar with printed medical journals, feed our entire coin collection into the library's photocopier, spend time on the Internet, consult with another doctor for an eleventh opinion, have long conversations with family members or close friends, call women we've never met who have had breast cancer, and still not feel confident about what treatment to choose.

Along with treatment decisions comes a new set of spiritual considerations. We may wonder if God plans to heal us—and if he does, whether he'll do it through treatment or "on his own." As we ask God to show us what treatment to choose, we may wonder also whether he'll respond, and if so, how we'll recognize his responses.

## If God Wants to Heal Me, Should I Listen to My Doctors?

A woman in her thirties who was diagnosed with breast cancer refused treatment because she was convinced that God was going to heal her without any help from medical doctors. Tragically, the woman died, leaving her children motherless and other family members and friends in shock and grief. What's even more tragic is that countless other women have died unnecessarily for the same reason.

Those who forsake conventional medicine to trust God for healing are motivated by a variety of convictions. One person may dismiss medical science and technology as humanistic, convinced that God doesn't approve of them. Another person may believe that God has personally revealed to her his plan to heal her without any help. Another person may assert that the only way that God can be glorified through her is by healing her miraculously and that she would be displeasing God by turning to medical science for help.

Is it wrong to trust God alone for our healing and not turn to conventional medicine? Are the two mutually exclusive? Bonita, who was diagnosed with breast cancer in 1989, was acquainted with the woman who had died while waiting for God to heal her. Watching the woman die raised the question in Bonita's mind about trusting God for healing, and she drew some of her own conclusions:

I knew from the beginning that God could heal me by whatever means he wanted to use. If he wanted to heal me without my having any kind of treatment or surgery, I felt like that would be revealed at the proper time—so that if I went back to the doctor prior to surgery or prior to chemo, and they said, "It's gone, and we don't need to do anything," then that would be God's way of healing me. But if I didn't hear that from the doctors, then I felt like I was to proceed.

I've always felt that the Lord wants us to do everything that we can in "the natural." And when we do that, then he does what needs to be done in the spirit. God gives us responsibility in life, and we don't just pray about everything and leave *everything* to him and we do nothing. God has blessed us to have the power of choice, he gives us wisdom when we ask for it, and he directs us.

My own feelings about trusting God for healing were similar to Bonita's, but my struggle was in whether I would hear God clearly if he tried to tell me that he planned to heal me miraculously. I deeply feared that after my surgery God would reveal to me that he had already healed me but that I hadn't paid enough attention to get the message in time to save my breast.

To assuage my fear, I mainly prayed. Every day. And asked my friends to pray. I also invited a few friends over to my house to pray with me. And that was immensely helpful. Although none of us ever received a message from God that he planned to heal me miraculously, God reassured me that whatever he wanted to say to me before I committed myself to the surgery, he would speak it loudly enough that I would hear him.

God didn't heal me miraculously. He healed me, at least temporarily, but he required me to lose my breast in the process, just like hundreds of thousands of other women. However, I'm grateful to him for choosing to heal me that way, because I've had many opportunities to tell others what I went through and how God was with me. If he had healed me miraculously, I'm not sure that many people who are not followers of Christ would have listened to me and believed me; even medical professionals often pass off such events as, "Sometimes these things just happen, and we don't know why." But because I am now identified with other women who have lost a breast, people I meet nearly always respond openly to my story.

It's important that we ask God to guide us even after we've chosen our treatments. Margaret, for example, stopped her chemotherapy after two rounds. Based on evidence that her breast cancer had already spread to several other parts of her body, her oncologist's prognosis had been that the chemotherapy would likely do nothing more than prolong her life by a few months. And Margaret was already spending those additional months trying to cope with the side effects of the treatments. So Margaret and her husband decided, after discussing the pros and cons, to stop the treatments and trust God for whatever he had in mind for Margaret's future.

Within the next few months, God intervened in the spread of Margaret's cancer. Her pain decreased dramatically, and for several months the results of blood tests were almost within the normal range. Margaret did not assume that the improvement was permanent, but she accepted it as a gift from God for however long he wanted it to last. And she did her part by keeping herself as healthy as possible—for example, by eating raw fruits and vegetables processed by a juicing machine to maximize her intake of nutrients. So the decision to stop the chemotherapy seemed to be the right one for Margaret. But does she recommend that other women with breast cancer stop their chemotherapy or avoid it altogether?

> I believe that God expects us to use the medical help available to us as long as there is hope of a cure. But with the hope of heaven, I see no justification for the use of extraordinary means to prolong a life that is almost over. Chemotherapy did not add days to my life. God did. But chemotherapy did stop the rampant growth of the cancer so that God could continue his work. I believe that God is sovereign. My life rests safely in his hands. I acknowledge that God can heal me. If he does, I want him to get the glory, not a juicing machine or a chemotherapy treatment.

Margaret emphasizes that she stopped the chemotherapy treatments because she knew that in her case they would not save her life. However, most breast cancer patients who undergo chemotherapy or another form of treatment choose to do so because they are told it will increase their chances of survival. Before choosing a treatment, we need to find out everything we can about what each recommended treatment can or cannot do. And we can thank God for making the latest technological and medical advances available to us. We can also pray, and ask others to pray with us, that we will make the best choices. And then we can trust God to help us make those choices.

### How Do I Know What God Wants Me to Do?

After we've resolved the issue of how conventional medicine may or may not fit in with our trust in God, we're left with the more specific question of knowing what God wants us to do.

For me, there were two issues. The first, which I described earlier, was how to find out whether God planned to heal me miraculously. The second was whether to have a mastectomy, as my surgeon and several other doctors had recommended, or to save an ounce or two of breast tissue (I had very little to begin with) by having a lumpectomy and radiation. My overriding concern was that I would not later regret whatever choice I made.

After I prayed for several days about those issues, I felt that I should schedule a mastectomy. I didn't feel that a miraculous healing was out of the question, however. So I scheduled the surgery and decided that if I later sensed God telling me that he was healing me, I would request another mammogram to verify that the cancer was gone. Meanwhile, I tried to keep my spiritual ears open, hoping against hope that my breast would be spared.

Most of the women I talked with followed a course of action similar to mine. They read about treatment options, they sought medical opinions from other doctors, they sought counsel from people they trusted, they prayed, they asked others to pray for them and with them, and they paid attention to whatever nudgings they sensed God was giving them. When they made their decisions, they felt peace afterward, which they interpreted as God's approval of their decisions. All of the women seemed to agree with Sherin's advice: "We should seek God first in everything we do. He makes all things possible, and that includes treatment." Bonita adds, "What we need to do is hear from him and be open—'Lord, order my steps so that I go the way that you want me to go.'"

Margaret found her decision process to be straightforward. She says she had excellent doctors who readily answered all the questions that she and her husband asked. Based on the medical advice and the reading they had done, the two of them then asked God to give them discernment.

I've always had a basic belief that God gave me a brain for a reason and that, assuming I've prayed about it and asked for his direction, he'll help me to understand the next right thing to do. And I've concluded that if I struggle more and more and get more and more confused, that confusion is probably from Satan; God, I don't think, ever wants to hide the right thing from us. So I did my homework, I prayed about it, and I chose certain treatments because they seemed the right thing for me. It was a purely individual decision; because of my age and my life circumstances, it was what I felt I had to do.

Through all the intricacies of treatment decisions that she and her husband needed to make together, Margaret saw God repeatedly answer the "Help me, Jesus!" prayer that she had prayed when she was diagnosed.

Sherin was told by her oncologist that chemotherapy would decrease her chances of recurrence by only 10 percent. As the result of "lots of prayer and faith in God," Sherin concluded that 10 percent wasn't worth destroying her good body cells. She turned it down and "decided to go with God's one hundred percent." That was in 1991, and so far, Sherin has been just fine without any treatment beyond surgery. She's happy that she apparently heard God correctly.

Margo regrets that she didn't take more time to get further medical information. She feels that she could have made a more informed decision, even though ultimately it may have been the same decision. Diagnosed at Christmastime, she rushed into surgery, but she now wishes she had put it off for two weeks so that she could have continued celebrating the season with her family. "It was the most horrible time on the face of the earth to try to deal with it," she says. As a mother whose children were young at that time, she had anticipated the pleasure of watching them enjoy Christmas. And as a former Young Life leader, she had looked forward to attending a national Young Life conference, scheduled for January; she had already purchased her airline tickets. But scheduling surgery right away, followed immediately by chemotherapy, meant that she had to cancel all her Christmas celebrations and travel plans.

Margo, who is large-breasted, also regretted that she had immediately chosen to have a mastectomy. "I was lopsided," she says. "I couldn't walk straight for a while; it was like I'd lost an arm. So I thought, *Why didn't I think about lumpectomy?*" Although Margo later realized that she probably still would have chosen a mastectomy because she had an aggressive form of cancer, she wishes she had been given time to choose carefully.

As we gather information about what treatment to choose, we subject ourselves to an onslaught of statistics that can scare us further and discourage us. Yes, we want to find out all we can, so that we can make informed decisions. But it's also important that we don't read or hear more than we can handle emotionally.

Even positive statistics are often not helpful. They might help us to determine what kind of treatment would be best for us, but they can be discouraging if we're looking at them to give us hope. For example, if we find out that we have an 80 percent chance of surviving our type of breast cancer, we're likely to worry that we'll be among the 20 percent who don't survive.

It's difficult, of course, to judge whether certain information will be helpful to us or detrimental when we don't know what the information is. A good guideline is to go ahead and read any handouts that our doctors give us and any general literature about breast cancer from the American Cancer Society, the National Cancer Institute and other cancer organizations. Such literature is not designed to scare us or give us more information than we need. We can find out from our doctors what kind of breast cancer we have and what our treatment options are, and we can look for information related to our situations. Then it's important to try to avoid reading or hearing any statistics about survival and any news items that don't relate to our kind of breast cancer. That means being on our guard when we're near a TV, radio, magazine or newspaper. It may also mean occasionally stopping friends in mid-sentence to question them before they tell us what they recently read or heard about breast cancer. We may find, by screening the information that assaults our senses, that our fear about dying of breast cancer decreases.

When we've been told we have cancer and we're flooded with emotions and questions, it's possible to make quick decisions that we'll regret later, especially if our doctors and others are telling us what we should do. The best way to avoid regret is, first, to seek God. We can lay out all our fears and questions before him and ask him to lead us, step by step, to the best possible decisions. Next, we need to get additional medical opinions, read up-to-date, scientifically based information about our options and seek counsel from people we trust—all the while continuing to pray and asking others to join us in praying that God would lead us in the process. He is a compassionate God who knows us intimately and wants the best for us. When we depend on him in our decision making, he helps us to choose what is right for our individual needs.

**How Does God Feel About Reconstructive Surgery?**

Those of us who choose to have a mastectomy must also choose between having reconstructive surgery and living with a scar in place of a breast. But the decision may not stop there. If we decide to have reconstructive surgery, should we have it immediately or postpone it for a while? And what kind of reconstruction should we choose—surgery using artificial substances or surgery using our own bodies? Within each category of choices is a further set of choices. Along with choosing our treatments, we need God to help us with these many decisions as well.

But how does God feel about reconstructive surgery? And if it makes no difference to him, how do we make the wisest decisions? Certainly we can start by inviting God to guide us in every step of the decision-making process. And then we can examine the most obvious issues.

First, we need to determine how we might feel with a scar versus "reconstructed" breasts. Not knowing exactly what we would look like can make the decision difficult, but most plastic surgeons who perform breast reconstruction can show us before-and-after photo albums of some of their patients who have undergone reconstructive surgery. After seeing those photos, we might find it helpful to stand bare-breasted in front of a mirror at home and imagine the type of scar across our chests that our surgeon said we would have if we choose not to have reconstructive surgery.

Second, we'll want to gather as much information as possible from reliable sources. Medical libraries and women's health resource centers provide literature about the pros and cons of reconstructive surgery. Armed with questions about the various techniques and their risks, we can then discuss our options with a surgeon. In addition, talking with other women who have had mastectomies can give us a sense of reality about what it might be like to live with a scar or with a "reconstructed" breast.

Third, we can talk with our husbands if we're married, and involve them in our decision-making process. It's important that they understand the risks associated with the various kinds of reconstructive surgery as well as we do and that they understand our desires. It's also important for us to discover whether we're basing our decision on what we want for ourselves or on what we think someone else expects of us.

Of the ten women I interviewed who had undergone mastectomies, only Nancy had had reconstructive surgery. Two other women are considering having it someday, but even they aren't entirely uncomfortable with their scars. And the seven others—eight, counting me—have no regrets about deciding against reconstructive surgery, just as Nancy has no regrets about deciding in favor of it. (Two of the eight, Viola and Sarah, have had both breasts removed.) Several of the women emphasized, however, that they were glad they had researched the subject and had talked with others about it, as well as prayed about it, so that they could feel confident in their decisions.

The married women also emphasized, without exception, that their husbands were completely supportive and wanted to leave the decision to their wives. Listening to their comments, I remembered with pleasure what John had said to me when I was considering reconstructive surgery: "I don't like the idea of foreign objects being implanted in your body, or the idea of your muscles being fiddled with. Although if it's something you need to do for yourself, I'll understand. But don't do it for me." I had been leaning toward not having reconstructive surgery, because of the risks involved, and God used John's words to reassure me that I was making the best decision for myself.

While the Bible doesn't tell us that we should or should not undergo reconstructive surgery, it does tell us that if we belong to God, his Spirit lives in us (Rom 8:11). Therefore, we can honor God with our bodies by valuing them as he values them. For some women, that means having reconstructive surgery—perhaps because they don't want to look at a scar where a breast used to be, they wouldn't feel normal otherwise or they would simply feel better with a normal-looking breast. For other women, it means accepting a scar as part of their bodies. No matter what we choose, if we have invited God to be involved in the process, we can be assured that he will help us.

# 6

## FACING TREATMENTS & THEIR SIDE EFFECTS

Whad happens during treatment of our breast cancer can mean the difference between whether we live or die. Yet, while we're willing to do whatever we can to save our lives, survival may come at a high cost. Every kind of treatment poses additional risks to our health and well-being, and we may be required to suffer pain, sickness or fatigue for several months, as well as be left with fears about the harm that might be done to us over the long term.

God knows all of the short-term and long-term risks of our treatments. Although he doesn't guarantee that we won't have to face them, he does promise to be with us throughout the treatment process and afterward. If we believe that promise, we can face every aspect of our treatment, expecting him to make his presence known to us.

### Facing Our Fears About Treatments
We're likely to feel fear or dread as we face treatment, whether it's surgery, radiation, chemotherapy, oral medication, or any other means

of treatment. We might also begin to doubt that we've chosen the right treatment or the right timing of the treatment. Or we might be afraid that the treatments won't help and that we'll feel half dead from the side effects and then die anyway, having lost our last chance to feel normal.

So we're faced with the tension of wanting treatment in the hope that it will help us survive breast cancer, yet fearing the treatment process or the side effects or both. We might therefore experience, within the same hour or the same moment, both hope and fear or other conflicting emotions. Gerry experienced these roller-coaster emotions before and during her radiation treatments. "Sometimes I felt optimistic and confident, and sometimes I was agitated in spirit and frightened," she said. "And it went back and forth." Margo wanted to start her chemotherapy treatments as soon as possible after her mastectomy, because she was anxious to get rid of any remaining cancer cells. But she dreaded the treatments.

Rachel also dreaded the side effects she would likely face from her chemotherapy treatments. But she found a way to prepare for them.

> I knew I had this long one-year stretch before me. However, when Robert and I talked about that year's procedure, I said, "I was ill for nine months with all three of my pregnancies—just throwing up—and it was like walking through life with this little dark cloud following me. But once I gave birth, I was fine; it lifted." And I said, "Well, I endured twenty-seven months of nausea; I think I can handle another twelve."

I dreaded my own treatment, even though it would be over within a few hours rather than in six months to a year. I dreaded all the unknowns: the lack of control I would feel in being put under the anesthetic, the nausea upon waking up, the potential pain, the disrupted sleep, the scar, the grief, the limited mobility for a while, along with all those dark unknowns that hover in our thoughts without taking recognizable shape. My dread was somewhat diminished whenever I reminded myself that those things were not unknowns to God; he knew what he was leading me into. I found comfort in some words from Isaiah:

> But now, this is what the LORD says—
>   he who created you, . . .

he who formed you . . . :
"Fear not, for I have redeemed you;
  I have summoned you by name; you are mine.
When you pass through the waters,
  I will be with you;
and when you pass through the rivers,
  they will not sweep over you.
When you walk through the fire,
  you will not be burned;
  the flames will not set you ablaze.
For I am the LORD, your God,
  the Holy One of Israel, your Savior." (Is 43:1-3)

That passage of Scripture reminded me that although God won't keep me from experiencing pain and suffering, he will be with me and will protect me from more than I can endure.

Judy, a children's librarian, had been afraid that she wouldn't be able to tolerate radiation because of her chronic illnesses.

As I drove to a park for a children's program, I was feeling overwhelmed by the "what ifs" of radiation treatment. *What if it triggers a flare-up? What if I'm too exhausted from the treatments to work? What if the treatments lower my blood count?* As these thoughts were playing repeatedly in my mind, God reminded me of the verse I'd read that morning—2 Timothy 1:7. I was reminded that God has given me a spirit of power, not of fear; that the Lord is the Lord of my "what ifs."

Judy endured the radiation treatments without any side effects other than increased fatigue. And she was able to continue working.

Fears about treatment are real, and we need to pay attention to them. No amount of telling ourselves to be strong or to not be a crybaby will work for very long. But when we acknowledge each of our fears to God, he may surprise us with his responses.

## Experiencing God in Sickness, Pain and Fatigue

Sometimes the side effects of treatment can be overwhelming, and we have difficulty coping with them. But those difficult times may give us opportunities to experience God in new ways. Viola has had a variety of treatments, including several series of chemotherapy, for her recurrences of breast cancer. She describes what she often does when she feels overwhelmed:

> There are times when I feel that I just want to be left alone. I don't want any more needles either putting something in or taking something out, no more scans, no more X rays, no more hospitals, exhaustion, nausea, pain. My reactions have been anything from ignoring the pain, because I had to keep up with my house as well as work, to just lying down and having a good cry. Sometimes I would curl up in the recliner chair and try to get comfortable. Perry holds me when I feel this way and lets me cry. We both know that when I've cried all I need to cry I will pick up the pieces and continue on, because it's not up to me to tell God how much I can take.

Viola believes, however, that God understands her feelings.

> God and I had many talks about the pain, and he always let me know that he really did understand, that there was nothing I would undergo that he hadn't already experienced. What a comfort to have a heavenly Father who really understands! After all, he experienced a very painful crown of thorns, nails in his hands and feet, a sword in his side; he knows loneliness, for he was alone in the wilderness for forty days; and he felt rejection when his disciples turned their backs on him. Any emotion or physical pain I could ever experience he knows; therefore he will hold my hand through anything.

Judy often felt frustrated by the weakness and fatigue that resulted from her radiation treatments and compounded her chronic illnesses. But she was encouraged when God reminded her, she says, that he would be her strength (Ps 84:5) and that his "power is made perfect in weakness" (2 Cor 12:9).

Margaret vividly remembers God helping her through a siege of excruciating pain before she and her doctor discussed the amount of medication needed for controlling the pain.

> I think that pain is the one area where God is the only contact. Others can't help. It's the time when you're driven to God, because no one else can touch it; it's a very personal thing. For me, the pain would come twelve to fifteen times a day, in an intensity that was unbearable. *Unbearable.* And I found myself back to that primitive "Help me, Jesus" prayer in the middle of the pain, where no one else could reach me, where it was a matter of trying

to survive the second and then the minute. And I found that God was faithful there, to get me through that minute and then that next minute and then that next minute. He was there with me in the pain and eventually brought me through it directly. I don't know that I've ever been or felt so primitive. Pain reduces you to such a place of simplicity that survival is the only thing relevant. And I was so aware of God's presence.

On one of those days of unbearable pain, Margaret received a gift from God.

I was in my bedroom and noticed that the sky was black, but on the other side of the house there was sunshine. And I thought, *That's the formula for a rainbow.* And there was a light sprinkling of rain. So I looked into the clouds, trying to find the rainbow.

I didn't see it at first. And then I saw the faintest hint of a rainbow. There wasn't color, really; there was just a very faint outline of a rainbow. And so I started thanking the Lord. [*Tears come to her eyes.*]

Then a little bit of color came. So I thanked him for the color. And it got brighter. So I started praising him. And it got brighter still. And I started thinking, *Lord, what's on the other side of the rainbow? I know you are on the other side of the rainbow.*

Then it became a *double* rainbow. And I was overwhelmed with the generosity, the abundance, of his love for me. I was on my knees, praising him and crying. That was *my* rainbow! I know that hundreds of other people saw that rainbow that day, but it had *my name* on it. It was his way of encouraging me in the midst of my pain. And it was the most powerful evidence of the hope that I have in him—the fact that when I see him, he's going to be on a throne with the colors of the rainbow. And all of who he is will be fully evident to me then; I'll be able to see it. It was such a powerful message, such a gift!

God has not promised us freedom from sickness, pain, fatigue and other side effects of cancer treatment. But he has promised us that he will be with us and will show us his infinite love.

### Experiencing Depression During Treatment

If you've ever been sick or in pain or physically exhausted for weeks on end, you probably wondered if you would ever feel healthy again. Perhaps you lost hope and became depressed. Although not every woman who is undergoing treatment for breast cancer experiences depression, it is a common response.

Margo describes her treatment stage as darkness. "It was *all* dark. In my head, I knew that God would be with me and bring me through it. But it was a very dark time." Nancy, Jane and Judy also experienced darkness in the midst of treatment. Nancy says that she avoided buying new clothes, because she didn't know how long she'd be around to wear them. Jane says she found herself reading obituaries—that she was unable to shake the "darkness" that surrounded her, even though she had never before experienced depression. And after Judy's mother died of cancer, Judy thought, *Why bother continuing the treatments? I'll probably die from cancer soon too.*

When we're in the midst of darkness, we may find it hard to pray. We yearn for God more than ever before, but the words don't come, and sometimes all we can do is fall on our faces and cry in his presence. That was true for Gerry when she was feeling worn down by weeks of radiation treatments:

> There are times when your prayers taste like cardboard and you don't feel that anything you're doing or saying has any real effect. You don't feel spiritual, and your prayers don't come out right, and you're absorbed in yourself. I cried when I was sad or hurting or exhausted or discouraged. Sometimes I found that to be very refreshing; I could get the emotions out and *then* pray.

The prophet Isaiah understood that darkness. "We look for light, but all is darkness; for brightness, but we walk in deep shadows" (Is 59:9). God does not intend for us to remain in darkness. He tells Isaiah, "I will turn the darkness into light before them and make the rough places smooth" (Is 42:16). The prophet Micah was confident of that promise. "Though I sit in darkness, the LORD will be my light," he wrote (Mic 7:8). And David proclaimed in one of his psalms, "My God turns my darkness into light" (Ps 18:28).

But sometimes such words can sound like nothing more than words. Sometimes we're not even sure that God is there.

### Has God Abandoned Me?

Joan had never experienced depression. But although she had followed Christ since her youth, she felt distant from God following her recurrence, and she later realized that those feelings had turned into depression. "I felt very dry and deserted, like God had left me. I cried a lot. And when I was by myself, I would scream and holler at God, 'I don't understand! Why are you doing this to me?'"

Not truly believing that God had given up on her, Joan didn't give up on God. Throughout the six weeks or so that she felt abandoned by him, she earnestly sought God by reading from the Psalms. She identified with many of the feelings expressed by the psalmists, and as she prayed those prayers herself, she began to again recognize God's presence with her.

> David experienced so much of that anguish. And I felt it was OK for me to experience all this. I was allowed to; I didn't have to feel guilty. And through the Psalms I could read just how much God *did* come back. I would know his presence again, and I felt his warmth coming back. I started to feel *myself* come back again.

Also during that period Joan was studying the book of Job in a group Bible study. Job's declaration "Though he slay me, yet will I hope in him" (Job 13:15) became Joan's anchor while she felt distant from God. She began to view that sense of distance as a way that God was stretching her faith in him.

> I learned in these trials we face that we have a choice to make. And that's whether to believe that God is there or to tune him out. It's scary to be thinking, *This is a time when I don't want God any more; I don't think I need him.* I wasn't believing it, but I think I was entertaining it and wondering. And then I really did come to my senses and think, *No, even though I don't feel all the warm fuzzies, I* know *he is there.*

Job, King David and Jesus himself serve as models for us when we feel that God has abandoned us. In Psalm 22 David cries out:

> My God, my God, why have you forsaken me?
>   Why are you so far from saving me,
>   so far from the words of my groaning?
> O my God, I cry out by day, but you do not answer,
>   by night, and am not silent. (vv. 1-2)

Obviously David wasn't ashamed of feeling that God had abandoned him. And he didn't hide his feelings from God, even though he feared that God wasn't there to hear his cries. Jesus, as he agonized on the cross, quoted David—"My God, my God, why have you forsaken me?" (Mt 27:46)—and yet Jesus was "without sin" (Heb 4:15). If Jesus' cry was acceptable to God, then we also can freely cry out to God when we're afraid that he has abandoned us. Crying out to God is an expression of faith, even when we're afraid that God has broken his promise to always be with us. We are acknowledging to God and to ourselves that something in our hearts won't let us stop believing in his goodness, no matter how we feel. God might allow us to feel abandoned by him for a time so that all that's left is our simple faith that he is with us.

### Seeing Our Treatment as an Ally

It's a double irony that when we feel perfectly healthy we could have a disease that might kill us, and then the very thing that's supposed to help make us healthy feels like it's killing us. Perhaps before our treatment began we were already seeing our bodies as a battleground, in which our healthy cells were defending their turf against the invading cancer cells. If so, it's hard to understand how any treatment that makes us feel worse could be anything but another enemy, pummeling us until we're too weak to fight back. We're told that feeling awful can be part of the process, and yet when we're in the midst of throwing up or we're sprawled across our beds unable to lift an eyelid, our perspective can become as blurred as our vision.

The time may come when we need to choose between seeing our treatment as another enemy or as an ally. Several of the women I interviewed remember making that choice. Rachel, whose chemotherapy was partly oral, had always felt anxious as she popped her pill each morning.

> One morning I got up and ate breakfast, and then I knew that when I took the Cytoxan I was going to become ill. But I looked at that little pill and thought, *God has provided this for me as healing, and that's what I'm accepting it as. This is going to be an act of obedience every time I do this.* And that turned it around for me; I lost the anxiety. That struggle had been

making it really difficult, but I began to accept the medication as God's gift of healing for me.

Jane took a Walkman with her to her chemotherapy treatments and discovered a song that helped her to see her treatment as an ally.

I played it over and over, because it was the way I pictured what God was doing in me. It's a song that John Denver sang, called "The Flower That Shattered the Stone."[1] And I always pictured Christ as my "flower" that was coming in and shattering all those cancer cells.

Some of the women found that reciting Scriptures to themselves during their treatments helped them to see their treatments as their ally. Bonita meditated on Mark 16:18 during her chemotherapy treatments: "When they drink deadly poison, it will not hurt them at all"—because, as Bonita says, "that's what chemo *is;* it's poison, and it kills your cells. And I'm praying, 'Lord, let it kill the bad cells and not the good cells.'"

When we anticipate undergoing treatment for breast cancer, we can ask God to give us some Scriptures or mental pictures to reassure us that our treatment is an ally, not an enemy. If we ever feel that our treatment is more than we can bear, we'll want all the reassurance we can get.

## Experiencing God During Treatments

Our God, whose imagination is infinite, has many ways of turning our darkness into light. Obviously he uses Scripture to help us understand who he is and what he has promised us. But in addition, he often uses songs, images, a sense of his voice or his presence, and answers to our prayers to dispel the darkness and fill our hearts with light.

During her treatment phase, Rachel found that the book of Psalms, especially in the modern paraphrase *The Living Bible,* was an anchor that kept her from drifting away from hope. Three weeks after her surgery, when she was still afraid that she would die of cancer, she came across Psalm 61:6-7: "You will give me added years of life, as rich and full as those of many generations, all packed into one, and I shall live before the LORD forever." Rachel made a note in her Bible that "if I lived a year, God's promise was that it would be as rich and full as those of many generations."

Bonita identified with the chronically ill woman who had faith that she could be healed by merely touching the hem of Jesus' robe (Mt 9:20–22). And Bonita found that the Scriptures strengthened her not only to endure her treatments but also to help others.

The Bible is full of help for us. It paints pictures for us and spells out the truths we need to hear when we're undergoing treatment—especially the truth that God loves us and is with us every moment.

Joan experienced God through a song as she woke up from her first breast surgery. The song was based on Psalm 42:1, "As the deer pants for streams of water, so my soul pants for you, O God." Joan was surprised to find that her husband, George, had been humming the same song during her surgery.

Several of the women sensed the presence of Jesus in the room with them when they were undergoing their treatments or resting at home between treatments. Jane had a bone scan performed, on the advice of her doctor, and as she was overhearing the concerned comments of the technologists attending her, she became afraid that they were seeing something that meant she would die. In the midst of that fear, she sensed Jesus standing next to the table on which she was lying. Although some of the fear stayed with her until she found out that the bone scan was negative, she felt comforted by a continued sense of Jesus' presence.

Although some of the women sensed God's presence without any effort, others found comfort by intentionally picturing God or Jesus in some way—or picturing themselves with him—and focusing their attention on that picture during their treatments. Gerry chose to picture herself "as a little child, resting my head under the shadow of his wing." Because she felt "hurt and scared and wounded," she was comforted by that image.

When Judy underwent her simulation procedure, in which she was "tattooed" and measured for future radiation treatments, she had to lie with her arms over her head for an hour and a half.

> Because I was in the midst of a fibromyalgia flare-up, this was a very painful position for me. When I didn't think I could keep my hands over my head another second, God brought to my mind a vision of Christ

hanging on the cross—the agony caused by the position of his body on the cross, especially the position of his arms. I realized that he, who had suffered so much more than I, understood my pain. With this picture in my mind, my remaining time on the table was much easier to bear.

Some of the women talk about hearing the voice of God during or prior to treatment. For me and for several others, his voice took the form of a mental impression, or that voice inside us that is quieter than a whisper and that we know isn't us. I often experienced God's voice in that way in response to my prayers, as I sat still and tried to listen to him with an open heart. Sometimes he gave me a Scripture passage to meditate on or a Scripture reference to look up. At other times, he reassured me—not always by quoting himself—of his presence and his love.

Bonita describes the first and only time she has heard the audible voice of God. Her husband, Carl, was driving her to the hospital for her lumpectomy when it happened.

I was quiet and subdued. Then I heard God's voice in my ear, saying, "Fear not, O daughter. I go before thee. The battle has been fought and the victory won." The tears started rolling down my face, and my husband looked over at me—"Are you OK? Everything's going to be all right." And I said, "No, it's not that. God spoke to me." I grabbed a piece of paper and a pencil, and I wrote it down. And I wrote down that it was at 10:40 a.m., September 27, 1989.

When I'm saying it was audible—no, Carl didn't hear it, but it was as though God had whispered it into my right ear. He might as well have been—and I guess he *was*—sitting right there next to me and saying it to me. I was overwhelmed with that message, that God was going before me, and I took that in terms of the surgery, that I didn't have to worry and he was going there. And then "The battle has been fought and the victory won" was in terms of my illness and that I had the victory in all this. It's as real now to me as it was then. That voice—I've never forgotten how real that felt.

And you know how you check into the hospital and they put you into your little gown on your bed and you don't have anything with you? [*She holds up her hand and closes it tightly.*] But I held on to that paper, and when I went into surgery, I had it in my hand. They had started to put me under the anesthesia, and the doctor came into the room and said, "What's this in your hand?" And I said, "Oh, no! [*She looks intently at her closed hand.*] You can't take this; this is my *word!*" And he said, "OK, but we'll just put it over here, and we'll give it back to you."

I told my mom about it later, and she said, "You know, I was praying that you would hear from God yourself." I had heard from different people, "You're going to be all right," "Everything's going to be fine," "We're praying," and that's a comfort to hear from other people. But to hear from *God!* There's nothing like hearing from God.

Bonita later printed the message from God in large letters, framed it and hung it on her wall, where it has continued to help her. "I've always drawn on that word," she says, "that if God said that I had the victory in this, well, it wasn't just for that day; it was for this whole cancer experience."

The rest of us may never hear the audible voice of God while we're still on this earth. But we can take comfort that our God is a communicative God, one who will go to almost any length to tell us what we need to hear when we need to hear it. Whether we receive the sound of his voice as explicit words in our ears or as a vague impression in our minds, we can be assured that he cares for us enough to communicate with us.

God has promised to supply all our needs "according to his glorious riches in Christ Jesus" (Phil 4:19). This promise includes the special needs we have as we undergo treatment for breast cancer. When we open our hearts to him, he gladly comes to us and meets our deepest needs.

# 7

---

# RESPONDING
# TO CHANGES
# IN OUR BODIES

As much as we want to believe that beauty, in the common usage of the word, is only skin deep and that true beauty is far deeper, we still tend to think of a beautiful woman as one who has, among other attributes, two breasts and a full head of hair. So when we have to lose one or both breasts and perhaps our hair and undergo other physical changes that disturb us, our beliefs about beauty are severely tested. We don't even feel normal, much less beautiful. Is beauty—or, in our case, what we perceive as normality—less important to God than we thought? How does he see us, with our bald heads and our scarred, flat chests? And can he help us to feel normal, or even beautiful, once again?

Our God is a God of beauty. He created beauty, he loves beauty, and he personifies beauty. But he does not define beauty as the world defines it. He sees us as beautiful, even in our hairlessness, breastlessness, weight gain or loss, permanent "tattoo" from the radiation, teeth discoloration, and any other changes in our bodies. He does indeed, as the women in this book testify, help us to regain a healthy body image, in which we can see ourselves as beautiful. And as we begin to see ourselves the way he sees us, we see more of *his* beauty.

### Losing a Breast

The attitudes of women about having to lose a breast are as varied as the breasts themselves. For some, it's a huge adjustment to accept their new shape; others view it as almost a nonevent, considering that their lives are at stake. One study has shown that women whose breasts play an important part in their appearance or in their sexual relationships are likely to have more difficulty in adjusting to their loss of a breast than women who place less importance on their breasts.[1]

I found it interesting that most of the women I interviewed who had had mastectomies didn't find it difficult to give up their breasts. And although Nancy is the only one who has undergone reconstructive surgery, all of them say they adjusted quickly to the changes in their bodies. The consensus seems to be that these women had enjoyed having two breasts but that they were much more concerned, at the time of their surgery, with getting rid of the cancer than they were with what it might be like to have a scar where a breast used to be. And after their surgery, they were focused more either on surviving chemotherapy or on feeling relieved that the cancer had been removed. In addition, these women say that their breasts had never been central to their sexual identity. The married women were fortunate to have supportive husbands who continued to love them and affirm them after the mastectomies were performed. The married women also reported that their sexual relationships with their husbands were not at all hampered by their loss of a breast. (The effects of breast cancer on our sexual relationships are discussed further in chapter eight, "Reaffirming Our Sexuality.")

Of the women I interviewed who had undergone mastectomies, several grieved over the loss of their breasts, but all of them eventually began to accept how they looked and understand that God saw them as whole. Here are what a few of the women said about their experiences:

> I was satisfied with my womanly shape before the mastectomies; I had reconstructive surgery after my mastectomies. However, I never felt

diminished in any way because I no longer had my own breasts. (Nancy)

In the end, I felt thankful that I didn't have a lot of my identity tied up in my breasts. (Jane)

I suppose that what the Lord did for me was that he put people around me that just thought I looked great. Every time someone would see me, they would say, "Oh, Connie! You look wonderful!" And I used to think, *Well, what did you think I was going to look like?* I never asked them, but I stayed healthy-looking. That was nice of the Lord to do that. (Connie)

The loss of my breast was a separate trauma from having cancer. I grieved the loss of my breast. But God sees us as whole, and this body is only temporary. I have my life, and my faith in Christ is strengthened. (Sherin)

Sarah had struggled with her sense of femininity ever since finding out, at age seventeen, that she had only tiny specks for ovaries. Being told in her forties that she needed a mastectomy renewed her struggle for a little while.

I was shocked. I was feeling rather unfeminine already, being infertile and not being like other women, with the monthly thing. I'd had the estrogen to promote some breasts, and here I was, going to *lose* a breast. When it came to the actual day, I was a hopeless mess. I thought, *I used to wear a bra with cotton in it, in my teens, and here I am—I'm going to be going back to that again.* And I thought it was a bit ironic, really. But I think what God was saying was, "You're not going to be any less feminine with just one breast." I was reassured by that.

Sarah was among those who adjusted quickly, which was especially fortunate because of what happened to her later. Only a year and a half after her original diagnosis, cancer was discovered in her other breast, and Sarah decided to have a second mastectomy. She seemed, however, to be at peace with that decision, even long after the surgery and despite her choice to not have reconstructive surgery. Again, as with most of the women I interviewed who had mastectomies, Sarah has been more concerned about saving her life than about losing one or both breasts.

It's hard to know exactly how we'll feel about the loss of a breast before it happens. Before her surgery, Viola had had no problem accepting the loss of her breast. But as she lay in a hospital bed recovering from the surgery, she wondered if the reality would prove harder than the anticipation. The night before she was to have her bandages removed, Viola shared her concerns with God.

> I basically said, "God, I'm a little apprehensive as to my reaction when the doctor removes the bandages. Let me feel your presence." The next morning when I awoke, before I even opened my eyes, God said to me, "Just remember, Viola, that I see you as perfect." It was so real and audible, that I opened my eyes expecting to see God standing beside my bed. I was sure that Marge, my hospital roommate, must have heard him too. The doctor came in, removed the bandages, and really, it was no problem and has not been since that time.

God chooses many ways to reveal himself to us when we seek him. Although most of us don't hear his voice audibly, we can recognize his presence in other ways. In my own loss of a breast, I experienced God in a way that was intimate and personal.

My difficulties in accepting the loss of my breast are rooted in puberty. As my breasts began to develop, I looked forward to having breasts like my mother's—or at least something that approached cleavage. However, by the time I was twelve, after barely getting started, my breasts stopped growing. Considering that I already felt handicapped by my translucently pale complexion and "skinny" frame—a combination that sometimes led teachers, school nurses and my peers to label me as sickly or weak—my attitude toward my body was in trouble. It wasn't that I wanted to be like Raquel Welch, whose bosom was the cultural ideal during that era; I just wanted to look normal, never mind the cleavage. And to me *normal* meant that I should at least fit into an A-cup bra without space left over. So throughout my teens, in the privacy of a locked bathroom, I often looked down at my chest and cried. I begged and pleaded and argued my case before God that he should order my growth hormones back to work and not allow further damage to my already low self-esteem. But my breasts never budged.

When I began to attend ballet performances as a young adult, I noticed that the female dancers onstage had chests like mine. Yet I was captivated by their beauty and sophistication. Slowly I began to feel confident that I looked feminine, sleek and attractive, just like the female dancers I admired. And eventually I thanked God for giving me small breasts.

So I felt betrayed when, at age forty-one, I found out I would have to give up half of my meager endowment. It had taken me about twelve years to accept my breasts as they were—small, but a matched set—and now it seemed that I was going through the experience all over again. I kept telling myself that I should be glad to give up my breast rather than die of cancer. But I was heartsick nonetheless. And as I lay on the operating table awaiting the mastectomy, I was not comforted by the surgical nurse who opened my gown and squealed, "*Oo-ooh!* You're so *small!*"

I alternated between scanning my mental files for sarcastic comebacks and dutifully blessing my persecutor. But in the midst of those thoughts, I sensed a strange peace, once again, about giving up my breast. And I knew it was from God.

I had talked with God, both before and after the surgery, about my feelings of betrayal. I wasn't angry at him, because I was fully convinced that he loved me and that he gives us only good things. But I was angry that I had to lose a breast. And I know he listened to me. Even before I knew that the "atypical cells" in the mammogram were cancerous, I sensed God telling me that he was taking me on a long journey that would be full of new adventures and that he would be very close to me throughout the journey.

Over time, as I held on to that promise, God replaced my anger with hope. He spoke to me through reassuring Scriptures, through panoramic views of mountain ranges, through the quietness of my heart and through the compassion of my husband and my friends. And God made me feel loved. I soon realized that although I was missing a part of my body, I was now closer to wholeness than I had been when I had both breasts.

But the journey hasn't ended. After nearly eight years, my old prosthesis looked like it was about to lose its goopy contents through its frayed edges, so I went shopping for a new one. I also decided to try once again to find an authentic mastectomy bra—a bra with a built-in pocket—so that I wouldn't have to keep pinning a separate pocket inside my comfortable, all-cotton seven-dollar sports bras. But after an hour of trying on itchy, lacy forty-dollar mastectomy bras and being told by the prosthesis fitter that she would have to order a size 0 prosthesis (which might still be too big, so that I end up having to buy a lumpectomy prosthesis, as I did last time, even though it wasn't an exact match either), I headed for the escalator, fighting tears. I was hearing the same not-quite-spoken message I'd heard when I had shopped for my first prosthesis: *You're just too small.*

So I was surprised an hour later when the shopping trip ended happily. Having arrived at the mall hoping to buy a prosthesis and a bra, I waltzed out to the parking lot with new running shoes and sunglasses. Did it matter much what was under my blouse as long as I felt comfortable and sophisticated? Maybe my old prosthesis was about to deflate, but my self-image wasn't.

God doesn't see us as one-breasted (or no-breasted) women. He sees what's on the inside. We, however, are affected by what we see on the outside. But God cares about how we feel about our breasts, and he can help us see ourselves as he sees us.

## Losing Our Hair

Feeling the water from the shower sloshing around her ankles, Margo looked down to see why it hadn't drained from the tub. But before she could discover the cause, she was shocked to see that the tub was now black.

> Can you imagine a white tub turning black? I couldn't see the bottom. I thought, *What in the world is going on?* And I realized it was all my hair. I'd washed my hair out, and it floated everywhere.
> I sat down in the tub and cried. I thought, *Well, this is it; here I go.*

The timing was ironic. It had happened in a hotel bathroom while Margo accompanied her husband to a medical meeting (he's a medical doctor) to get her mind off her chemotherapy treatments.

Margo's only warning that she was about to lose her hair was from her oncologist, who had told her she *could* lose it. For some women, it never happens; for others, it happens gradually. Joan, for example, had to vacuum the bathroom floor two days in a row after blow-drying her hair. The next time she washed it, she "sort of knew" that the rest would be coming out. "George stood there with me while my hair was falling out as I washed it," she says. "And I was crying. Then I looked at myself in the mirror and just about freaked out. It was so scary, so frightening." Joan was comforted, however, by the presence of her husband.

Viola, who underwent chemotherapy five times in fifteen years, lost her hair every time. "I probably had more trouble with the loss of hair than I did the loss of the breast," she says. Her hair grew back in gradually, so that it was all different lengths. She also found, like several of the women I interviewed, that her new growth of hair had a different texture. Some women who had straight hair found that their new hair was curly; others found that their new hair was coarser. However, if you've lost your hair because of chemotherapy, take heart; any change in texture is usually temporary.

What kind of head covering to wear, if any, is a big question for us when we're facing chemotherapy. We might not lose our hair, but what happens if we do? Talking with those who are close to us about losing our hair can help us see ourselves in healthy ways. When Margaret lost all her hair, she discussed with her husband how he felt about seeing her bald head, how *she* felt about her bald head, and whether she should keep her head covered when they were at home alone.

> He said, "It doesn't bother me, except that it makes me feel so sad, because there's a verse in the Bible that says a woman's hair is her glory." And he said he felt so sad that chemotherapy had taken away that glory. Then he said, "It doesn't bother me to see it. But for your own dignity, I think you ought to wear a hat or scarf of some kind." So that's what I do. We were able to talk about it and come to a mutually satisfactory solution. It wasn't something uncomfortable. I felt perfectly free to ask him what he thought, and he felt perfectly free to tell me. That means a lot.

When we're able to talk with those who are close to us about what to wear over our bald heads, we give them an opportunity to reaffirm who we are. We also give God a chance to help us regain a healthy attitude toward our bodies, so that we feel confident when we go out in public, no matter what physical changes we've experienced.

Sarah had been advised to buy her wig before starting chemotherapy, because the scalp can become sensitive once the hair begins to fall out. So she invited a couple of friends to go wig shopping with her, which turned a dreaded chore into a small party. Sarah was grateful also that her friends thought of questions to ask the salesperson about the wigs that hadn't occurred to her. She knew that by buying the wig in advance she would be wasting her money if her hair didn't fall out. But her hair did fall out, and she was happy with the wig. "I got tons and tons of compliments," she says.

When I first met Elena, I was struck by what beautiful, healthy hair she had, which was cut in a flattering pageboy style. It wasn't until later that day, as we talked about the effects of her chemotherapy and she lifted the top of her hair two inches to reveal her bald head, that I realized I'd been fooled by a wig. But then she surprised me again by telling me that her eyelashes as well were not her own. She had lost her eyebrows and eyelashes in addition to her hair. "One day I thought, *The sun is hurting my eyes. There's something wrong.* And later I noticed I had lost my eyelashes. It was so fast."

Elena was fortunate that her wig and false eyelashes looked natural on her and that her scalp could tolerate the wig. But of course she looked forward to getting rid of them. When I saw her again a few months later, her hair was about an inch and a half long all over her head and most of her eyelashes and eyebrow hairs had grown back, even though she was scheduled for several more months of chemotherapy.

Sometimes our hair doesn't grow back until well after the chemotherapy treatments are over. But whenever it happens, it's cause for a celebration. Joan, having finished her chemotherapy treatments in November, was about to spend Christmas Day cooking, when she decided to reveal what had been cooking under her hat. "I had everybody coming in for dinner," she says, "and I thought, *I am not cooking and wearing a hat.* So I took it off, and my hair was pretty short. But it was the official time-to-take-the-hat-off day, and I never wore the hat again." Joan appreciated her family for making her feel normal with so little hair on her head.

Losing our hair seems like a gross injustice when we already have been subjected to the indignity of baring our breasts to what may seem like the entire health care community. But it's often a necessary evil.

And God can help us to remember that we are beautiful and that we are loved—by him as well as by our families and friends.

### Responding to Other Changes in Our Bodies

Losing our breasts and our hair are not the only physical changes that we might experience during treatment. For example, surgery, especially breast reconstruction, can mean limited mobility and soreness (both of these are usually temporary); chemotherapy drugs can discolor our teeth and cause us to lose weight or sometimes to gain weight; and tamoxifen may result in a dry throat and changes in weight.

Jane was shocked to discover she had gained twenty pounds after starting to take tamoxifen; she's only five-foot-one and had never had a weight problem. After going on a low-carbohydrate, high-protein diet, however, she is now back to her original size and "feeling like myself again" while continuing to take tamoxifen. Margo gained fifteen pounds after starting on the drug, and although she's considerably taller than Jane, she was dismayed that she was never able to lose the weight. She stopped the tamoxifen after five years—the recommended length of time for taking it—and immediately lost the extra pounds.

Sarah, however, lost a lot of weight during her most recent chemotherapy series. Although some women have teased her with comments like, "Oh, you *poor thing*. Such a *problem!*" she wasn't happy about the weight loss. Her previous weight was about normal for her five-foot-seven frame, and she feels somewhat self-conscious about looking thin. She smiles contentedly, though, as she reports having gained back a few pounds.

Although we each know that we haven't changed on the inside, physical changes, especially the ones we never wanted, can make us afraid that other people will see us differently. But we can know that God still sees us as beautiful. "I am fearfully and wonderfully made," said David (Ps 139:14), who sometimes cried out to God that he was being shunned by his friends and neighbors (see Ps 31:11). God does not belittle our fears about looking different. When we cry out to him about such fears, he responds with his love, so that we can eventually see our bodies the way that he sees them.

If you're facing chemotherapy and have been told you may lose your hair, here are some suggestions that might be helpful:

■ Talk with other women who lost their hair during chemotherapy. Hearing them describe their experiences, even with all the negative aspects, may help you to feel less alone.

■ Consider cutting your hair very short. If it falls out, you're likely to experience less trauma if you're already used to seeing less hair on your head.

■ Ask someone in your oncology department to refer you to a wig bank that provides wigs and hats to cancer patients at no charge. If no one there knows of one, check your local Yellow Pages under "Cancer." If no wig banks exist in your area, contact the nearest chapter of the American Cancer Society for help.

# 8

---

# REAFFIRMING
# OUR SEXUALITY

W e naturally feel apprehensive about the prospect of sexual intimacy after we've had breast surgery or other treatments for breast cancer. Whether we're now missing a breast (or both breasts) or the affected breast appears damaged, we wonder how our husbands, or our future prospective husbands, will respond to us. And whether we're married or not, we might also find it difficult to see ourselves as sexually whole following surgery or during treatment. Several questions may arise in our minds: *Will I be just as sexually attractive now as I was before the surgery? Will my ability to function sexually be affected? Will my scar—or anything else about me—inhibit sexual satisfaction for either my husband* [or *my future husband*] *or me? Will I have no choice about remaining single? Am I sexually something less than I was before?* Or, *Will my marriage be over?*

Although we've all heard the horror stories of women who had mastectomies and then were deserted by their husbands or boyfriends, those situations are the exceptions. Relationships that are going to break up when the woman has breast cancer tend to show signs of trouble long before the mastectomy is performed. Among the married women in this book, the experience of breast cancer instead drew their husbands closer to them.

The closeness that we might experience—or, for single women, perhaps the hope of closeness in a future relationship—is often preceded, however, by some emotional struggles that can last from a few days to a few years. The questions that we ask are real, and we need God to help us find the answers.

### Feeling Less Sexual

God created us as sexual beings. He has given us the gift of sex within the confines of marriage as a means of finding mutual pleasure and satisfaction with our marriage partners, as well as for the purpose of procreation. (See the Song of Solomon, as a vivid example, in which the bride is "faint with love.") So when we begin to feel less sexual— whether it's due to the chemicals being used in our treatments, to the loss of a breast, to a feeling that we're less attractive or to a combination of factors—we may begin to wonder if we will ever become fully sexual beings again.

Rachel, who was forty-five when she was diagnosed, remembers struggling for a little while with her sexuality, because of the chemotherapy drugs. "I felt dead," she says. "I had no responses, and it was really hard." And Joan became concerned, after her mastectomy, about how her sexual intimacy with her husband would be affected. Even now she sometimes avoids looking at herself in the mirror when she's undressed.

For a single woman who is being treated for breast cancer and is committed to staying sexually inactive while single, doubts can arise about attracting a potential mate and finding sexual fulfillment, if she has had such hopes. Judy, who has never been married, was relieved that she didn't have to have a mastectomy, because chronic illness and a recent hysterectomy had already left her "feeling like damaged goods," and the fear of a mastectomy reinforced those feelings. Although she wasn't dating anyone at the time, she wondered "if the stigma of cancer would scare guys away." Viola is certain that if she had still been married to her first husband when she had her first mastectomy, he would have left her. When she had to lose her second breast, she occasionally thought, *I guess I'll be single the rest of my life. What man would want someone with both breasts missing?* And Sherin, who also was divorced, felt "mutilated" following her mastectomy and began to hope that any future prospective husband would see her and love her "from the inside out."

Those of us who are married find ourselves looking to our husbands for some of the answers to our questions about our sexuality. It's vital that we talk with our husbands about our questions, even if we're afraid of the answers we might receive. Talking with a close friend or a counselor can also be helpful, whether we're single or married. But we need more than the answers we find through those who are close to us. We need *God* to respond to us.

### Experiencing Depression Related to Sexuality

Sometimes during treatment our questions and our fears about our sexuality can so overwhelm us that we become depressed. The depression can be fleeting, or it can last for months or even years beyond the treatment process. Two of the women in this book, Margaret and Joan, say they experienced depression when their sexual drives were lowered as a result of chemotherapy. Although they both knew that their depression may have been chemically induced, it was nonetheless real. Joan was surprised by it, because she had had chemotherapy once before and her sexuality hadn't been affected. But this time she was getting stronger drugs, and she faced new side effects. "I'd lost a lot of interest in sex," she says. "I felt very ugly—no hair, and feeling low because of the chemo. It was a very difficult thing to deal with. I did not feel attractive at all. That was my biggest problem. And I felt very bad for George."

Chemotherapy treatments can cause not only a temporary decrease in sexual desire, as in Joan's case, but in some cases also the onset of temporary or permanent menopause. And decreased sexual desire can result from menopause. When Margaret first had breast cancer in 1988, her chemotherapy treatments put her into sudden and permanent menopause, at age forty-two. Hit with all the symptoms practically overnight, she felt devastated, and she became angry.

> Anger was really raging. I was angry at God, because I didn't feel feminine or sexual, and I felt that I had lost a big chunk of who I was. I didn't know

how to express the anger, and I just turned it inward. It was like a whole big part of me had been chopped off and I was supposed to keep going on. I still had this career I wanted to pursue, and yet the part of me that really mattered had been injured. I felt that even though I had won the battle of breast cancer, it had really won in the long run, because it had taken a big part of who I was.

Margaret might have benefited from talking with a trusted friend about what she was experiencing. But the thought of doing so was more than she could handle at the time.

It seemed almost unreal, as if there isn't really anything to talk about but something's really wrong and I don't know what it is. People didn't understand where I was; *I* didn't understand. I felt like I was having to reinvent myself. I felt like I was alone and I didn't have anybody to talk to about it. Chuck didn't understand; it was impossible for him to understand. And it wasn't something I could talk about with others. Maybe I should have gone into therapy; at one point I thought about it. I had lost interest in life, and yet I had a business to run.

Margaret credits God for bringing her out of the depression. She had avoided God because she was angry at him, but she feels now that he has turned her heart away from blaming him and toward loving him again.

As he did with Margaret and Joan, God wants to make us whole. Whether we're married or single, he wants us to see ourselves as whole beings, sexually and emotionally, not as anything less than how he designed us. For example, when Jesus met the Samaritan woman at Jacob's well, all her sexual and emotional heartaches were supernaturally revealed to him. Jesus treated the woman with compassion, offering her "living water" (Jn 4:10) that would satisfy her forever, whether she remarried once again or remained single. This "living water" describes our relationship with him, in which we can daily draw on his love.

Some Christians spiritualize this passage, saying that the intended purpose of this living water is to take our minds off sex and other supposedly worldly values and fill them with "spiritual things." But we mustn't oversimplify the application of this Scripture by dismissing all our normal desires, including sexual desires. I believe that Jesus' metaphor of living water—a never-ending, rushing stream—also signifies the fluidity of our relationship with him. That is, we can have ongoing dialogue with the one who created us as sexual beings. We can ask him questions about whatever may be disturbing us sexually, we can tell him our fears related to our sexual needs, and we can cry out to him, even in anger, if we're depressed over our sexuality. While crying out to God doesn't usually result in the immediate disappearance of the depression, it's a vital first step.

### Recovering Our Sexuality

Although our sexuality can be violently threatened by treatment, we can fully recover, sexually and emotionally, even if the "package" isn't the same. God himself, through the Bible and his personalized care for us, can help us see our bodies and our sexual needs from his perspective, while he also uses our friends and husbands to firmly root us in the confidence that we can be sexually whole.

Sometimes the questions we might have asked about how our breast cancer treatments will affect our sexuality are answered before we have time to ask them. This was true for Joan. But she tried to do something about her lost sexual drive. After she recognized some of the causes of her depression she felt free to focus on the love that she and George had for each other, rather than on how she looked and felt physically.

> That was something that I really had to work through, and yet it was so amazing that George would tell me, "I still love you the way you are; I don't care." And I would say, "But I'm so ugly—no hair and I've got this stupid little thing on my head." It amazed me what true love is, that he could just put all that aside; it didn't matter to him. And I thought, *Wow! I've got myself a gem.*

Despite her lingering struggles with looking in the mirror, Joan knows that her husband's feelings for her haven't changed. "It was a process for me to allow myself to feel whole around him," she says, "whereas he never saw it as a problem. I think it brought us much closer. When we were intimate, it was very good; he was very loving. You realize that wholeness comes from within." Joan's ability to focus on the relationship itself, along with her reassurance from George, enabled her to relax and feel less inhibited sexually. Her depression soon lifted.

Joan's process of feeling whole again was helped along when a friend gave her a framed passage of Scripture to hang on her wall. The passage, from Psalm 139, describes how intimately God knows us, with such statements as, "I praise you because I am fearfully and wonderfully made" (v. 14). Joan describes her response to the gift: "I thought, *Yes, I am created by God and am very beautiful.* So God made me feel like, Yeah, it's all OK—that I'm still a very worthwhile person and that even when I'm feeling like this, he still loves me very much and I'm right there in the palm of his hand. He understood all my needs."

For those of us who are married, our husbands can be our main source of help in regaining our sense of sexuality. Close friends can be instrumental as well. Margaret tells how a friend helped her to feel attractive to her husband again:

> Exactly ten days after my lumpectomy, a woman in our church called me and said, "At four o'clock this afternoon, I want you to go take a nice, long, hot bath, put on your sexiest nightgown, and set your table with your nicest china. I'm bringing you a gourmet dinner."
>
> She brought a basket filled with a five-course dinner—chicken *cordon bleu* and all this wonderful stuff, including a fancy little dessert—and she said, "It's time that you are a woman again. You're not a cancer patient tonight." And I thought, *How very wise of her.* She had waited just long enough for me to start feeling better after the surgery and start realizing that I still am a wife and I still need to be intimate, and she provided the stimulus that I needed, to take my eyes off myself and focus on my husband and have a good time.
>
> And it was wonderful. It was such a gift from God, for getting back on track sexually and remembering that even though we've been scarred we're still very capable of intimacy. And it's a nice break from having to deal with the cancer—to focus on the comfort that sexual intimacy can give. It reminds us of what's really important.

God was involved in my own experience of sexual loss from the beginning. There was never a question in my mind that John hadn't married me for my breasts. (At a size AA, they weren't one of my prominent features.) And I wasn't seriously worried that he would lose interest in me sexually because I now had only one breast. But if I had any unconscious doubts, they dissolved a few hours after I'd had my bandages removed, when he examined my scar, looked tenderly into my eyes and said, "I still think you're beautiful and sexy."

Even now, nearly a decade later, I occasionally feel ugly and misshapen. But I always find comfort in John's words, because I know he still means what he said. His reassurance was not an isolated burst of sympathy for his traumatized wife.

That is not to say that I didn't have some adjustments to make sexually. Like many women whose recovery proceeded well, I found that a subtle, unsettling feeling chafed at my heart like a foxtail in my sock—the kind of thing that makes one feel guilty for being bothered by it. It was an effect of the mastectomy that I hadn't expected: the loss of sensation. I was about 80 percent numb from just below my armpit to where my nipple used to be. Having been told to expect some temporary numbness around the scar and that possibly a fraction of that numbness would become permanent, I didn't let it bother me at first. But the numbness never went away, and I began to realize that most of my nerve endings, along with my breast, were gone forever. John didn't mind, but I did.

Although I still sometimes feel sad about the lost nerve endings, I can see how God has helped me to become content with my partly numb chest. The loss might have been a bigger deal to me if my breasts had been central to my sexuality, but God has reminded me through John that I'm a sexual being, not just a person with sexual parts. The result is that I now feel no less feminine, no less alive, no less attractive to my husband. And our sexual relationship, we agree, hasn't suffered one bit.

For Viola, God's process of restoring a sense of sexuality was even more gradual. Lying in a hospital bed after her first mastectomy, she felt stung when her ex-husband called and told her, "You've lost a very important part of your female body."

> I had fleeting thoughts in which I wondered if there would ever be anyone in my life or if the loss of the breast would make that impossible. But as I continued to work and carry out my responsibilities as a mother and homemaker, I realized I was no different than I was before. Besides that, when I would really get thoughtful about this, I was reminded of God's words, "Just remember, Viola, I see you as perfect." If God sees me as perfect, how dare I see myself as anything less?

Twelve years later, when Viola was being treated for a recurrence, she became friends with Perry, who had lost his wife to breast cancer. "He knew that I needed the support of someone who understood," says Viola, "and I knew I could call him if I needed to talk." Not until after Viola had her second mastectomy (and no reconstruction) did she and Perry have their first date. As they began dating regularly, Viola felt apprehensive because of her ex-husband's remark. She thought, *If losing one breast was that important to my ex, how will Perry feel about my not having either breast?*

When their relationship began to look serious, Viola said to Perry, "I know if I had still been married when I had my first mastectomy my husband would have left. This was something that he would not have been able to deal with." Perry responded, "So parts are more important than the person? It doesn't matter to me what you have or don't have. It doesn't change who you are, and it's *you* I love."

Perry doesn't feel that he had always been so compassionate, however. His first wife, who was only thirty years old when she was diagnosed with breast cancer, underwent a lumpectomy and then a mastectomy, and Perry wasn't sure how to help her except to let her know that the loss of a breast didn't change how he felt about her. Feeling frustrated and helpless, he became impatient with her when she had adverse reactions to her chemotherapy, and they often argued about what Perry now calls "the old male attitude." Perry had become "pretty much a workaholic," he says. "God was not really a part of my life at that time, and that's what really makes the difference."

As Viola's and Perry's relationship developed, Viola became further convinced that Perry was not concerned about what was missing from her body. He had lost part of his thumb when he was a child, and when Viola asked him about how he would deal with the fact that she had had a double mastectomy, he asked her how she would deal with the fact that half of his thumb was missing. "Good point," she said. Viola began to feel that she had nothing to fear in marrying Perry.

> After we were married, I was able to completely accept the fact that it really didn't matter that I have no breasts. I have never felt ashamed or self-conscious in front of him. He has had no hesitation in touching me,

nor have I in letting him touch me. Perry's complete honesty and total acceptance of me pretty much took away all doubts.

Viola and Perry were married in 1996, only a few weeks before Viola entered City of Hope Hospital near Los Angeles for a high-dose chemo/stem-cell (bone marrow) transplant. The bride was fifty-nine years old; the groom was fifty-three.

Sexual wholeness is no less real and attainable for single women who are undergoing breast cancer treatment than it is for married women. Because they don't have a husband as a potential source of sexual affirmation, they may need to rely more on close friends or a counselor to help them regain confidence about their sexuality. They may also need to consider at what point during a serious dating relationship to let the man know they've lost a breast or have suffered other permanent physical effects from the cancer treatments. God is concerned about all the fears we have about our sexuality, whether we're single or married.

Nowhere in the Bible does God say that a woman is incomplete without a man. In fact, as many of us used to hate (or still hate) hearing, celibacy is a gift that God gives certain individuals so that they can devote more attention to him and not be concerned with serving the needs of a spouse. And as Viola, Sherin and Judy have proven, it is possible, with God's help, to regain our sense of sexuality without a husband. For those of us who are happily married, one of God's purposes in giving us compassionate, understanding husbands is to reaffirm our sexuality. When our sexuality is reaffirmed, we can enjoy a closer relationship with our husbands. But whether we are single or married, allowing God to reaffirm our sexuality can ultimately help us understand how much God loves us and values us.

---

If you're looking for ways to help regain your sense of sexuality after breast surgery or during other treatment, here are a few suggestions. Most of them relate to married women, but if you're single, read them and take heart that you can feel sexually whole.

■ Tell your doctor about any aspect of your sexuality that you feel you've lost. If you're undergoing chemotherapy or taking other medication, your doctor may be able to identify the loss as a side effect and may have some suggestions. If your doctor prescribes medication, however, be sure to ask what side effects of the new medication you might experience, and then ask your pharmacist to let you read the package insert before you decide whether to fill the prescription. Also, ask God to help you make wise decisions.

■ Remember that hormone replacement therapy poses a risk of recurrence to women who have had breast cancer. Talk with your doctor about your options, such as nonhormonal vaginal creams.

■ Tell God your fears or other feelings about your sexuality. Remember that he cares about *all* your feelings. Be alert in the next few days and weeks for what he may tell you or show you.

■ Talk with a trusted woman friend about what you're experiencing. If you're married, talk with your husband about it as well, and discuss what the two of you can do that might help you. For further help, see a counselor, alone or with your husband.

■ If you've had breast surgery, encourage your husband to touch the scar as soon as possible after the bandage is off. During lovemaking, you may need to remind him that the scarred side needs love too.

■ Tell your husband specifically what still gives you sexual pleasure and what, if anything, to avoid. If he seems inhibited, he's probably afraid of hurting you. Encourage him to ask you questions and to express his concerns.

■ Ask your husband to list for you all the things he likes about your body and any other things that attract him to you sexually. Do the same for him.

■ Buy your husband a card that expresses your love for him, and leave it on his pillow.

■ If you like to write, consider writing an erotic poem or essay about your husband. Then surprise him with it when he's not distracted.

■ Discuss with your husband the possibility of setting aside a regular time to massage each other or to give each other a "love bath," with or without sexual intercourse. Being physically caressed, and physically caressing him, will play a vital part in helping you to feel more sexual.

■ Plan some romantic dates with your husband, away from home, whether it's a movie, a candlelight dinner, a stroll through your neighborhood on a moonlit night or a hike to the summit of your favorite mountain.

■ Do some spontaneous romantic activities away from home, such as driving to a romantic spot after dinner to watch the sun set or to gaze at the stars. While you're there, reminisce with your husband about how the two of you first fell in love with each other.

■ If you and your husband like to dance, put on a CD that you both like and invite him to dance with you. Include some long pieces that are good for slow dancing. Or plan a date for getting dressed up and going out dancing together.

■ Indulge yourself in whatever makes you feel like a woman. Take bubble baths. Get a facial, a manicure, a makeover, a new hairstyle or a professional massage. Wear comfortable but feminine clothes whenever possible, and save the baggy sweats for when you feel more confident about your sexuality. Wear a fragrance when you go out, when you're around your husband or when you're at home alone. Wear a sexy nightgown to bed, even if it reveals a missing breast or two.

■ Do whatever makes you feel confident about being a whole person. Take initiative in your home, your workplace, your church, your supermarket. Call friends. Follow up with business contacts, or help a coworker solve a problem. Visit someone who's lonely. Ask the supermarket manager why your favorite brand of frozen yogurt was discontinued. Doing these things won't affect your sexuality directly, but God can use them to remind you that others see you as a whole person.

# 9

# KEEPING OUR
# RELATIONSHIPS
# INTACT

Breast cancer is not a private experience. Our families and friends have their own shock to deal with, and the shock waves may continue throughout our treatment process. Those who are closest to us may be afraid of losing us, or they may be worried about how long we'll take to recover or how soon their lives, as well as ours, can return to normal. And others may feel awkward, not knowing what else to say to us besides "How are you feeling?"

About midway through the treatment phase is where our relationships tend to undergo the most rigorous testing. Friends, family members and acquaintances have already sent us cards and flowers, called us to express their shock and sympathy and assured us of their prayers. Our husbands—for those of us who are married and whose husbands are supportive—have listened to us and held us while we cried, and perhaps they have mopped the floors, prepared some of the meals, intercepted phone calls and taken the kids to karate lessons. And we've sat down with our children or grandchildren to tell them, as well as we can, what it means for us to have breast cancer.

During our treatment phase we may find ourselves occasionally wanting to help others respond to us. Although we're probably not at our creative and assertive best, there are some things we can do to help keep our relationships intact. And we may find that some of those relationships deepen as a result.

### Keeping Our Husbands Close

For some of us, having breast cancer doesn't dramatically change how we and our husbands relate to each other. But for others it can make a big difference. For example, after Margaret told Chuck that she was not expected to survive her recurrence, they decided to forgive each other for all their "petty hurts and grievances" and to love each other unconditionally. As a result, Margaret and Chuck immediately began to see a difference in their marriage. They agree that although their marriage was good before, their commitment to forgive each other—a pattern that they've continued—has made it better.

Like Margaret, Joan has no idea how to plan for the future, and she's concerned about the responses of her husband, George. She wants to hear about his feelings as well as tell him about her own. Wanting to encourage his wife, George sometimes interprets Joan's need to talk as a sign that she's given up hope of surviving. So Joan has a dilemma: she wants to accept George's encouragement to keep going, but she also wants to prepare him in case God doesn't heal her. "I believe that the Lord will let me know when the right times are," Joan says, "and that George will be ready to hear it." Joan and George occasionally find those times to talk, and Joan is committed to maintaining open, honest communication with her husband.

From the time that they hear of our diagnosis, our husbands' lives are shaken by our cancer. Their minds, like ours, are bombarded with questions: *Will she die? What would I do without her? How much will she suffer? Why is this happening? Am I equipped to take care of her and to comfort her? What can I do to help her? How will our lives be changed, and for how long?* Our husbands' fears naturally affect how they respond to us. And just as we need their assurance that they will be available to comfort us and support us, they need our assurance that we need them and want them. In addition to telling them, "I need you and I want you," we can help them by being honest with them about what we're feeling and by inviting them to share their feelings with us.

In a society that does not encourage men to face their feelings and talk about them, men tend to sweep their feelings under the mental rug of analysis and objectivity. When they see a problem, they want to be able to fix it and move on, detaching themselves from any possible fears and feelings of helplessness. Not being able to fix their wives' breast cancer leads some men to tell themselves and others that their wives are handling it just fine and there's nothing to worry about. And being invited by their wives to talk about how they feel doesn't immediately change them. Husbands may be concerned that expressing their feelings will upset their wives. And unfortunately, their wives, wanting to calm their husbands' fears, sometimes play the game by acting as if they are indeed doing just fine.

This game of denial, while making the husband and perhaps also the wife temporarily more comfortable, can ultimately divide them. The wife is left to deal with her feelings either alone or with someone other than her spouse. The same is true of her husband. And if they are not aware of their own feelings, they may soon see their feelings—or each other's feelings—arise in destructive forms, such as anger that is inappropriately expressed.

So what can you do to encourage your husband to lift up the rug and look at his feelings? Here are a few suggestions.

*Set an example.* Yes, our husbands expect us to express emotion because we're women, whereas men are supposed to be strong. However, you might draw out your husband by talking with him about your own feelings. When you identify some of your fears, you can ask him, "Does this scare you too?" You can help him to value his feelings by telling him, "I know this is hard for you" or "I know you're as scared as I am."

*Encourage him to talk by asking specific questions.* You might ask him, "Are you worried about whether I'm going to survive?" or "Are you afraid that you won't be able to give me the emotional support that I need?" If he says yes, ask him to describe his worries or fears.

*Tell him what you need.* You might say, "I need you to hold me, to tell me you love me, to listen to me when I want to talk, and to not try to talk me out of feeling bad." You might also assure him that he doesn't need to worry about saying the wrong thing.

*Invite him into every phase of your experience with breast cancer.* Don't try to protect him. Share with him everything you find out about your type of cancer. And ask him to go with you to your next medical appointment. Husbands usually want to be involved in their wives' medical treatments; it gives them the sense that they're doing something to help. And having that sense can sometimes free husbands to talk about their feelings.

In addition, you can tell your husband how much you value him. Invite him to pray with you. Discuss with him any past grievances that either of you are harboring, and then agree to forgive each other. If he doesn't respond to any of these suggestions, it may be that he's afraid and is trying to protect himself from pain or discomfort. His fears may surface as anger. Or he may withdraw from you. You might ask God to soften his heart, and then look for opportunities to share with him your own feelings, little by little. Keep telling him that you appreciate his presence with you and that you need him.

No matter how our husbands respond, our cancer experiences can strengthen our marriages. When we express to our husbands how much we value them, when we're honest with them about our feelings, when we invite them to participate and when we resolve any past hurts that have come between us, we give God the opportunity to use our cancer experiences to draw our husbands closer to us.

### Talking with Our Children and Grandchildren

Elena's heart sank when her three-and-a-half-year-old son, Michael, said to her, "Mommy, I don't want you to die. I *love* you, Mommy." Elena realized that although she hadn't told Michael that cancer is a deadly disease, he had somehow figured it out.

We dread seeing our own fears reflected in our children's eyes. We want to be strong for them, but if they cry, will we be able to hold back our own tears? How much do we tell them about our cancer and our treatments? What if they ask questions that we don't know how to answer? And what do we say if they ask, "Are you going to die?"

Children know when something is wrong, especially if it involves one or both parents. If they sense that their mother is seriously ill, they become terrified of losing her, and they look to her to alleviate their fears. Sherin, for example, reports that one of her young sons slept in a sleeping bag on the floor in her bedroom until he felt sure that she would be OK. But in addition to the fear of losing their mother, many children are also afraid of saying or doing something that will make their mother feel worse. So, unlike Sherin's son, they might withdraw into a dark place within themselves, perhaps believing that they did something to cause their mother's cancer or that she would be displeased by their fears.

The best way we can alleviate our children's fears is to talk with them about what is happening to us and invite them to talk with us about their feelings. When Jane told her twelve-year-old son and nine-year-old daughter about her breast cancer, her daughter asked the question that no parent ever wants to hear from a child: "Are you going to die?" Believing that her children would imagine worse things if they didn't know the truth, Jane responded, "Yes, I *could* die from this, but I don't believe I'm going to."

Right after Jane had her mastectomy, she explained to her children that she now had a thin, horizontal scar where her breast used to be. Her daughter expressed interest, so Jane showed her the scar. The daughter said, "Hey, you just look like *me* now." And they joked about how Jane's scar looked like an eye that was winking. Jane's son didn't seem interested in seeing his mom's scar, which was fine with Jane, but she was amused by his comment: "Mom, breasts are just not important anyway." Jane decided that her son's attitude was appropriate for his age, "and we had a nice conversation about what breasts mean."

Although we can make our cancer experience easier on our children by explaining to them what is happening to us and inviting them to ask us questions as they arise, we can't expect to relieve *all* their fears. Sometimes children act out their fears when their parents aren't around to observe them. Bonita anticipated that possibility with her two young daughters, so she met with their teachers and explained that she was sometimes sick following a chemotherapy treatment and had to "sleep away that first twenty-four hours almost." She told them that "if there were any issues—if they saw anything going on with my kids in school, any change in behavior or attitude—to let me know, because I couldn't always 'read' everything at home."

Apparently the teachers never observed any unusual behavior in either of the girls, but Bonita's mother, who often stayed at their home when Bonita was sick, observed that ten-year-old Erika often peeked around the door of her parents' bedroom to look at her mom. Erika seemed concerned about whether her mom was OK, and her grandmother often talked with Erika about what her mom was going through. Erika and her seven-year-old sister, Erin, did sometimes ask their mother, "How come you're in bed?" and "How come you're not going to work?" which told Bonita that her children were frustrated that their lives were still being disrupted by her cancer. She gave them simple answers: "Because you know Mama has to go to the doctor and get my treatment. And when I get my treatment, I don't feel well afterward and I need to sleep. But I'm OK."

Like younger children, our older and adult children may not know what to say or ask and may try to hide their fears. But we can draw out our older children by involving them in our treatment experience more than we might with younger children. Margaret, for example, invited her adult son to go with her to doctor appointments a couple of times when he was in town to visit her. He went, and he seemed glad for the opportunity to ask the doctor questions directly rather than always asking his mother.

Janaha, who was in high school when her mother had metastatic breast cancer, has some urgent advice for mothers: "Talk! Even if the teenage daughter or son is saying, 'I don't want to talk about it,' they need to. They *want* to." Janaha says she wishes her mother had explained to her exactly what was happening in her body and what the prognosis was in terms of surviving or dying, and even the fact that her hair might fall out during chemotherapy treatments. Janaha wanted her mother to prepare her for facing a hard situation and to reassure her that her fears were normal and acceptable.

> There were a lot of things that I felt afraid to feel, and I was very unclear on how I was supposed to *be*. I knew I needed *something* at that time; I just didn't know what I was allowed to need. Because she was my mother, I would naturally go to her, but I knew that she was ill and that she was dealing with her own things, and part of me was maybe a little scared to go to anybody else. The person I really wanted was my mother.

Occasionally Janaha observed that her mother was experiencing peace and joy once again. But that made Janaha even more hesitant to trouble her mother with her own feelings. Janaha says, "I remember thinking, *If I go to her and tell her I'm afraid and that I'm hurting and I'm depressed and I don't know how to 'do' this and I don't know how to 'be,' then that's going to make her get depressed and feel the pain again.*"

When Rachel returned home from the hospital after her mastectomy, she was concerned about what her children, who were in their teens, might be feeling. So she looked for an opportunity to relieve their fears.

> We were sitting around talking in the living room one night, after I had recovered enough that I had gotten my prosthesis, and the subject of my prosthesis came up. So I said, "You guys want to see it?" I pulled it out and tossed it to my youngest son. He held it in his hands and said, "Oh, so *that's* what a breast feels like!"
>
> We all laughed. Then I showed the kids my scar. I said, "This is what it looks like, and you know—it's OK."

Children of every age need us to invite them to talk about what they're feeling in regard to our cancer. Younger children, especially, tend to have layer upon layer of fears—everything from whether we're going to die and leave them motherless to whether we'll be out of bed to fix them breakfast the next morning. When we talk with our children, we need to be honest with them about our cancer.

When Connie explained her chemotherapy treatments to her grandchildren, they all cried together, Grandma included. But then, on Connie's suggestion, they gathered up her hair that had fallen out and put it outside for the birds to make nests from it. "God can use everything," Connie told them. As a result of her hopeful attitude, her grandchildren became more hopeful.

Because we're already trying to deal with our own fears about our cancer, we might feel daunted by the task of conveying hope to our children and grandchildren. Joan faces that issue every day. "As a parent, you want to protect them, and you don't *want* them to go through it," she says. "It is just a truckload. I can put myself on the back burner a lot easier than I can my family." But talking with them about our breast cancer and encouraging *them* to talk about it helps them to be hopeful. It also strengthens our bond of trust with them.

There are many things you can do to allay your children's or grandchildren's fears. Most of the suggestions that follow apply to young children as well as to older children who are still in the home. A few may apply also to adult children.

*Explain to them, in terms and amount of detail appropriate to their ages, what is happening in your body,* including what your treatments involve and what differences they might notice about your appearance or your behavior.

*Encourage them to ask questions.* And be honest and complete in your responses to their questions and comments, without burdening them with unnecessary medical details.

*Reassure your young children that they can't "catch" cancer.* Most of the illnesses that young children know about are contagious, so it's natural for them to believe that they might catch your cancer.

*Tell them that it's OK to feel afraid or frustrated or angry or disappointed or sad.* Invite them to talk with you at any time about their feelings, and encourage them to talk with other trusted adults—family members, neighbors, teachers or the parents of friends. First, check with those adults, to see if they would be willing to talk with your children if the occasion arises.

*Reassure them that you're doing everything possible to get well.* You'll want to explain that sometimes the medicines or treatments may make you tired or sick, but that after a long time, you expect to be OK again.

*Communicate hope to them.* You might tell them, for example, "I believe that God will take care of us."

*Reassure them that you love them and value them.* They may need to hear "I love you" or "Tell me what you did today" more often now. And even though you may have less time to spend with them, the attention you give them may become more important to them than ever.

*Tell them how you feel about God in light of your cancer.* Sometimes adult children, as well as younger ones, wonder if God is punishing you or them or your family. If you sense this fear, reassure your children that your cancer is not a punishment. Tell them how you perceive God in your situation. If you are receiving any comfort or reassurance from God, your children will probably want to hear that, even if they don't share your experience of God. Know that you are in a position to greatly influence how they perceive God.

*Explain to them that your cancer is nobody's fault.* Young children often feel responsible for everything that happens within their families, no matter how hard their parents may have tried to avoid any form of blame in their household. Also, if your older children have heard about lifestyle factors related to cancer and are wondering "what you did wrong," you might explain that most women (70 percent) who get breast cancer have none of the identifiable risk factors other than age and that no one can be sure what caused your cancer.[1]

*If you need to be hospitalized, prepare them.* Tell them exactly where and when you're going, how long you will be there, why the hospitalization is necessary, what will be happening to you, who will take care of them and whether they will be allowed to visit you. Reassure them that you will miss them as much as they will miss you. And if you're considering inviting your young children or grandchildren to visit you in the hospital, be aware that they may become frightened if they see you hooked up to several tubes. (An IV tube by itself may not scare them, however.) Talk with them, in advance and preferably face to face, about how the tubes will look and why they are necessary.

*Tell them what will change and what will stay the same.* If their dad or someone else will be preparing your family's dinner more often, or if you are too fatigued to continue driving them to soccer practice or if the traditional summer vacation has to be canceled this year, they'll want to know that as soon as possible. However, they will also want to know that you'll still admire their drawings, read stories to them, put Band-Aids on their wounds, listen to them and take them places, whenever you have the energy.

*Tell them what they can do to help you or how they can be involved in your cancer experience.* The youngest children can bring things to you when you're resting after treatment. Older children can take on additional household chores, screen phone calls and prepare meals. Adult children might be willing to drive you to some of your medical appointments. If you begin to lose your hair, consider asking your children to brush it for you and to help you gather any hair that falls on the floor.

Involving them in your experience can help them to feel more in control and less afraid.

*Invite yourself into their world.* Draw pictures with your young children or grandchildren—pictures of your family and pictures of new or frightening things (IV bottles or you wearing a scarf on your head)— and then respond to each other's pictures. Read storybooks together— humorous books and classics, as well as children's picture books about cancer (check your public library).

Children are most likely to talk about what they're feeling when they know they can ask questions and expect honest, reassuring answers without being embarrassed or criticized. The main goal is to open the doors of communication. If you've done this in the past with your children, they probably already feel free to ask questions and express their fears. If you haven't opened those doors before, take heart; it's never too late. If your children don't respond right away, you might try issuing the invitation every few days, being careful not to pressure them so that they feel they're disappointing you by not responding. It is vital to also share with them some of your own feelings, as a way of letting them know that feelings are important. But however the communication happens, you can look forward to a closer bond with your children as a result.

### Helping Other Family Members and Friends Respond to Us

Because Rachel knew that many people feel awkward around someone who has a life-threatening disease, she found creative ways of putting those people more at ease. Rachel and her husband had been leaders of the college department at their church, so when she remained in the hospital after her mastectomy, she was pleased to be visited by two of the college men.

> They stood there looking at me. And I knew they just didn't know what to think. I guess, prior to my breast surgery I thought that was the grossest surgery anybody could have; I don't know why. But if I knew someone who had had breast surgery, I would wonder what it looked like. So those poor guys stood at the end of my bed, and I said, "Hey, you guys, do you know what my chest looks like? It looks just like my back, only it has a zipper in it." They laughed, and I knew they were much relieved.

Finding humor in our cancer may not be easy; there's nothing funny about losing a breast or fighting for your life. But if we can eventually develop a positive attitude—sometimes after slogging through a lot of difficult feelings and receiving God's compassion toward us in the midst of them—our positive attitude can take the form of humor, which can put others at ease and help them respond to us.

People may act awkward around us for many reasons, but they do so usually because they're afraid. The outcome is that they don't know what to say to us, beyond asking how we're feeling (and some people don't even do that). When Connie lost her hair, some people didn't know what to say to her. When her hair began growing back, they still didn't know what to say. Gerry, too, observed that some people neither talked to her about her cancer nor let her talk with them. Or those who mentioned it would quickly change the subject. And some who wrote notes to her used euphemisms rather than the word *cancer.*

We can't help everyone who doesn't know what to say to us. Gerry says, "I had people turn away because they either didn't know what to say or didn't want to be involved with my personal pain, physical or emotional. So I can't help those people." Gerry felt that she had enough to do in taking care of herself and in trying to encourage communication within her own family.

Gerry had not felt free until a few years after her cancer experience to tell someone close to her (not her husband, fortunately) what she had needed to hear from him during that time.

> I said to him, "You didn't talk much with me during that period, did you?" He said no. And I said, "You probably didn't know what to say," and he agreed. I told him, "The next time you have a situation with someone where you would like to offer comfort but don't know what to say, say *that.* For you to tell me, 'I would like to comfort you and help you and support you, but I don't know what to say,' *that* would have comforted me. It's honest, and out of that honesty can come further conversation. I felt scared, and maybe you felt scared too, but we could have taken it from there."

Gerry realized in retrospect some of the reasons that other people couldn't offer her any help: they felt awkward or afraid or helpless, or they didn't want to hear about someone else's pain. Yet we need our friends, family members and coworkers. So we have much to gain by trying to preserve those relationships, if we can expend the energy. It's important, therefore, that we determine which relationships should receive whatever attention we can possibly devote to them.

One of the first things we can do to preserve our relationships is to forgive those who have not responded in the ways that we wanted them to. Nancy, who was disappointed that some longtime friends didn't seem to understand her, says that it helped her to remember her own ineptness in similar situations. By putting herself in their place, she was more readily able to forgive her friends. When we've forgiven those who have hurt us, we have more strength for developing the relationships that we want to focus on, whether it's with those whom we have forgiven or with others.

Next, we can plan some ways to relieve any awkwardness that we have already observed or that might arise later. Rachel had anticipated the awkwardness of her college-age visitors, and she defused it by humorously describing her scarred chest. Frieda, a medical technologist, had "mini press conferences" with her coworkers just before beginning her treatments, because she didn't want any of them to feel uncomfortable around her. She explained to clusters of three or four coworkers at a time what was happening to her and then said, "You guys, I need you. I need your friendship, and I need you to talk to me. Hug me, or say something stupid, or make me laugh, but please don't ignore me." Connie found that some people weren't calling her, because they were afraid of waking her up. So she told them, "If I'm too tired, the answering machine will come on, but I need to hear from all of you. Feel free to call."

In addition, we can tell others specifically what we need. "I felt fragile, so I needed a lot of tenderness and expressions of love," says Gerry. "One doesn't want to be taken for granted—for example, 'Oh, we're friends, and of course you know all this, so I won't need to say it.' Yes, we *are* friends, but I *do* need for you to say it."

To maintain our important relationships, we can't always wait for those we care about to respond. Contrary to how we might feel, we may need to take the initiative. That means we need to talk, candidly and honestly, not only about what's happening to our bodies but also about how we *feel* about what's happening to our bodies. We need to use the word *cancer* and share with others our fears as well as our hopes. People who are waiting to pick up cues from us about how to respond want to know what it's OK to respond to. And if they know specifically what we're feeling, they are better able to respond compassionately.

# 10

## GRIEVING OUR LOSSES

R achel had accepted without question her doctor's recommendation of a mastectomy. Diagnosed with breast cancer in 1981, when treatment options were slimmer, her response was, "Get the cancer out of there. I don't want it in my body. And I'll do whatever you want me to do; just tell me." Later, she felt that she had handled the surgery pretty well emotionally.

But as she undressed one evening a couple of months after her surgery, she was caught off guard by some intense emotions. She sat down on the edge of her bed and began to cry—loudly. Her husband, Robert, heard her, so he went into the bedroom and sat down next to her. "Rachel, what's wrong?" he asked.

"Well, besides the obvious, I don't really know why I'm hurting," she said between sobs.

Robert, a hospital chaplain, had seen similar responses among many of the patients he had visited. And his words comfort his wife to this day: "Rachel, any time anybody loses a body part, they grieve. You've lost a really important part of who you are as a woman. And you're grieving."

Before we can recover from breast cancer emotionally, we must be willing to grieve all of our losses. Grief is not only a natural part of life; it is something that God values. We are told that God sets the times for us to grieve (Eccl 3:4) and that those who grieve are blessed, because they will be comforted (Mt 5:4). Jesus is described as "a man of sorrows, and acquainted with grief" (Is 53:3 KJV). And we are urged to grieve with those who grieve (Rom 12:15).

Grieving takes time. And not wanting to waste our time by feeling sad, we may try to avoid grief. Or we may not expect grief to be a part of our experience, and then we're surprised, as Rachel was, when our sadness suddenly erupts. When we take the time to grieve, however, we are acknowledging that something sorrowful has happened. We are facing reality. And facing our sadness by grieving gives God the opportunity to heal our hearts.

### Identifying Our Losses

We cannot grieve effectively until we are able to identify exactly what we've lost. For example, if we've lost a breast or part of a breast, it's obvious that we can grieve over losing a part of ourselves, but there may be additional losses we need to grieve over that are more subtle.

Judy was about to begin radiation treatments when her mother, who lived several hundred miles away, suffered a recurrence of lymphoma and was not expected to survive. Because her own treatments couldn't be interrupted, Judy had to decide whether to delay the treatments and visit her mother immediately or wait several weeks, until after completing the treatments, to make the long trip. Told by her mother's oncologist that her mother was doing well enough to survive another three months, Judy decided to begin treatments. But in the midst of those treatments, her mother died. So on top of suddenly losing her mother, Judy also had lost her last opportunity to see her mother alive. This continues to be an enormous cause of grief for Judy.

Margo grieved about having to cancel some family activities because she had felt rushed into having a mastectomy six days before Christmas. She also grieved about losing the opportunity to get a second opinion. Gerry grieved about losing valuable time, losing a sense of independence and control over her own life and losing certain friends who had either ignored her experience with cancer or ignored her altogether. And Margaret, who experienced menopause—suddenly, severely and permanently—at age forty-two, as a result of chemotherapy treatments for her first occurrence, grieved that she no longer felt like a normal woman.

Those of us who have had mastectomies have had several losses to grieve. Obviously, losing our breasts is the first reason we grieve; for some of us, that loss is traumatic. For me, it meant giving up half of what little breast tissue I had. For Sherin, who had her mastectomy at age forty-three, it was "like losing someone very close and grieving their death." For many of us, standing in front of a mirror and seeing a scar where a breast had once been became the norm after a shower or whenever we would change clothes. We may feel emotional pain from that scar for a long time afterward.

But we lose much more than the breast itself. First, there is the loss of sensation in the area of the breast—a loss that the finest of plastic surgeons cannot restore to us, even in the shape of a perfectly "reconstructed" breast. In a part of our bodies where we used to experience sensual pleasure, our nerve endings are dead. We now have numbness.

Second, we lose our normal, womanly shape. Sherin felt mutilated, and her grief over the way her body now looked affected her entire perspective.

> My life had changed, or the way I *saw* life had changed, and I couldn't go back to the old me. I couldn't *find* me. I felt I was on the outside looking in and that I would always have this nightmare in the back of my mind and be focusing on every little thing on my body.

Much like Sherin, Joan felt distorted and incomplete. She also felt jealous, at first, that other women had both breasts and she didn't.

> I think I looked at the breasts of every woman who walked in front of me. My eyes would zero in on women's breasts. I had to fight it so hard, because I didn't want it to be an obvious thing. And I felt ridiculous. But I thought, *They can wear different types of clothing that I won't be able to wear.*

If we choose to wear a prosthesis, as Joan did, our choices in clothing are limited. We have to buy special bras, usually at expensive department stores, or else sew or pin a special pocket inside each of our regular bras to hold the prosthesis in place. (This may require an extra few minutes for getting dressed.) We have to be sure when we try on new clothes, or when we put on the clothes already hanging in our closets, that the armholes of sleeveless blouses or dresses fit snugly, revealing neither the prosthesis nor the edge of the scar. If the prosthesis isn't the exact shape of the remaining breast—and it's hard for some of us to find one that is—we don't dare wear anything that fits tightly across the chest. Of course, low necklines are out. It's good-bye not only to the romantic evenings of revealing a little cleavage (for those who had it) but also to wearing loose-fitting, scoop-necked blouses. And just try finding a swimsuit with a high-cut neckline and cups that you can fit a prosthesis into. You probably would have to do what Joan and Margo did: go to a clothing store that sells mastectomy swimsuits and hope they have something in your size that doesn't look like what your grandmother used to wear. So, many of us, like Joan, might need to grieve that we have less freedom in choosing our clothes.

None of the women I interviewed were dissatisfied with their prostheses. But they do have their limitations. The greatest one is that they're merely part of our wardrobe; when the bra comes off, so does the prosthesis, and all we have underneath it is a flat area with a thin, pink scar. That reminder alone is enough for some women to grieve.

For a few of us, getting used to a scar across our chests isn't a big deal. It pales in comparison with the fear we felt about whether we would live or die, and we're relieved to be alive, breast or no breast. But after the fear of dying has passed, it can be helpful to examine every loss related to losing a breast and then determine how we feel. Many of us feel deeply sorrowful that we must choose between living with a scar and undergoing reconstructive surgery, between accepting a more limited wardrobe and facing the possible health risks associated with reconstructive surgery. These are all sad reminders that something life-threatening has happened to us and that we must live with the effects for the rest of our lives.

Those of us who had reconstructive surgery may have some different losses to grieve about. One is the loss of time that must be spent in surgery and recovery rather than in normal activities. Another is the nagging uncertainty about the possible loss of symmetry, because the new breast will not look exactly the same as the remaining, normal breast. And for those who suffer the tragedy of reconstructive surgery gone awry or implants that eventually leak, there might be a loss of health, as well as the loss of hopes for a normal-looking breast.[1]

Whether we've had to lose a breast or not, we may need to grieve also over the loss of certain assumptions about life. The assumption, perhaps, that we'll live to be at least ninety years old—and so will everyone we love. The assumption that, except for a rare disaster, life will be wonderful. And, probably the most subtle of all, the assumption that each disaster is only temporary and won't take long for us to "get over." If you never made those assumptions, then you won't have that loss to grieve. Or you may already have had those assumptions blown away by previous crises in your life. For some of us, however, it took getting breast cancer to realize that we had ever made such assumptions.

Margo remembers grieving over a "loss of innocence, a loss of the way life had been." She found that, although she had recovered from her cancer, she had to live with the possibility of recurrence. She often wonders *When is the next phase of it going to happen? When do we go around again?* For her, this loss of innocence was "huge."

Margaret has had even more to grieve about than most of us. Having received a diagnosis of terminal, she has had to give up her dreams. But she was not aware that she was grieving until she was well into the grieving process. What alerted her were certain things about herself that suddenly changed, such as an inability to carry a thought through to completion.

> My mind wouldn't work right. My problem-solving skills were right down the drain. To be confronted with something like reconciling a check-book, which I've done innumerable times and it's all on my computer—. All of a sudden I hit a snag, and I had to walk away; I couldn't cope with it.

Then Margaret noticed that she had lost interest in life. Often getting up in the morning without any agenda for the day, she began to wonder why she should get up at all. Then she noticed that she was feeling more emotional than she normally did; she was crying over things that previously she had paid little attention to.

Having received what she knew was the unmistakable peace of God about her diagnosis, Margaret was baffled by these sudden changes in her behavior. But she realized one day that she was grieving over the loss of her dreams. The dream of seeing the grandchildren that she hopes will be born. And the dream that she and her husband, Chuck, had shared of retiring in two years and living out their years in the Ozarks, the land of Margaret's roots. They had found some property that was everything they had dreamed of—sixteen acres, with a farmhouse, a spring-fed pond and six hundred feet of river frontage—at a price they could afford. Ironically, escrow had closed just two weeks before Margaret was diagnosed. She describes her grief over that loss while still in the midst of grieving:

> I don't have a clue why this happened. We were so confident that that property was God's leading. I love the country; I don't care for the city. And yet here I am, right in the middle of the city, and this is where I will be, unless God intervenes. So I realized that I was grieving over the life that I thought I still had, that I now know I don't have without God's intervention.

Although breast cancer does not mean, for most of us, that we have to give up our dreams, we can empathize with Margaret, because we tend to fear a recurrence. Also, we have at times wondered if we were going to live or die.

Our grief can have many raw expressions—tears, anger (including anger at God), the need to talk, silent withdrawal and thoughts about dying. We need to be sure that those expressions of grief are not harming us or those around us. For example, if I were to express my grief by silently withdrawing, John would wonder if I were angry at him. So I would need to assure him that my withdrawal had nothing to do with him. I would also need to try to talk with him about what I'm feeling, so that he wouldn't feel left out of my life.

In addition, we need to be sure that we're not rushing the grief process. Grieving takes time, and if we push ourselves to "get over it," we may instead push down the pain, only to have it erupt again when we're least expecting it. Stuffing our pain can have destructive consequences. Our bodies take on an extra load of stress, we lie to ourselves and to others and to God about what we're feeling, and we miss opportunities to grow closer to others and to God.

Allowing ourselves to grieve so that the grieving process does us some good means that we first need to identify our losses. Once we have done that, we need to allow ourselves to feel the depths of our sadness over those losses. Those two tasks, although difficult and painful, open the door for God to meet us and to heal us.

### Allowing God to Heal Our Grief

Some people believe that when we grieve our losses, we're not being "spiritually minded"; they may say we're weak in faith and that we're wallowing in self-pity. But they don't recognize that the Psalms are full of grieving. When King David and other psalmists cried out to God in desperation, they were not having a pity party. They were mourning; they were expressing genuine sorrow over something that had gone wrong. And God, in his mercy, heard their cries and answered them. David, for example, asked God to be merciful to him because both his soul and his body were "weak" with grief (Ps 31:9). Then he wrote,

In my alarm I said,
"I am cut off from your sight!"
Yet you heard my cry for mercy
when I called to you for help. (v. 22)

Just as David was not ashamed to ask God to comfort him in his grief, we can ask God to comfort us. And just as God comforted David, God promises to comfort us. "But you, O God, do see trouble and grief; you consider it to take it in hand" (Ps 10:14). God takes our grief seriously, and he does not reprimand us for grieving.

There are several helpful ways we can respond to our grief. One way is by crying; tears can help us identify what we're feeling. Talking extensively with friends or with a professional counselor is another way of responding so that we can receive God's comfort in our grief. Or we can journal about our feelings. Or we can pray—alone or with others. Some of us combine prayer and journaling by writing out our prayers to God, telling him specifically how we feel and asking him to comfort us, in addition to talking with others about our grief. I also found comfort—and still do—in sitting silently for a few minutes, meditating on God's love for me and waiting expectantly for God to speak to my heart or to increase my awareness of his presence with me. All of these responses to grief can be effective ways of receiving comfort from God.

Margaret still grieves over the loss of her dreams, and she's grateful that God is leading her through the grief process. He is helping her to identify, one by one, the specific things that she's losing. "But I'm not *overwhelmed* by the loss," she says, "and I think that's God's grace. He's giving me just enough grace when I can deal with it, and then a little bit more as I can deal with it." She also recalls that with her first occurrence of breast cancer, eight years earlier, she grieved over the permanent losses caused by her chemotherapy treatments. "So you don't have to be terminal to go through the grief process. When you've lost something that was a part of who you are, you grieve," she says, echoing Robert's words to Rachel.

Judy, who had prayed, journaled, and talked with her counselor about her grief over her mother's death, eventually found comfort in her strong belief that God was in control, even though she didn't understand his timing. Rachel found that the "little girl feelings" that she was grieving over matured into "maybe owning and embracing the prospects of death and of harshness in life and pain—embracing them in what seems like a healthier way." Sherin, who had felt mutilated and alienated from her own body, began to feel that her loss had become a gain. "When I look at the scar across my chest, I see God's grace," she says. And his grace got her through the grieving process, so that she was able to flourish. "I got over my grieving, got back on my exercise program, lost weight, cut my hair and bought a new wardrobe."

My own reactions to losing a breast were common to the experience of many other women, but the way that God met me in my grief was unique and personal. Despite having seen numerous photos of mastectomy scars, I was not prepared for what I saw when I looked down at my chest as the surgeon removed the bandage. I tried to admire the precision of the pink, pencil-thin diagonal line; it had no ragged edges or puckers. But I swallowed hard to hide my discouragement. My chest wasn't flat; it was *concave*. And the sight of skin stretched over ribs where I wasn't used to seeing ribs made me feel emaciated.

That evening, as I stood in front of the bathroom mirror after a shower, I wept. I felt ugly and misshapen. The area around my scar looked like a crater on the moon, and I hated knowing that unless I changed my mind and had reconstructive surgery I would look that way for the rest of my life.

As I cried out to God over the next several days, I was amazed at what he did. Feeling deeply grieved over the way I looked, I began to receive some hope and a sense of purpose from God about having breast cancer. I also began to feel joy over some good things that God was doing as a result of my experience. For example, my scarred chest reminded me that my body is only temporary—that it will serve me for only a few decades, and then my spirit will go to be with God, who will eventually give me a resurrected body designed to last forever. So I was glad to begin to see life as it really is: fragile and temporary.

One morning, still grieving, I prayed this prayer of thanksgiving:

> Father, I give you my entire body, including this "misshapen" portion. I give it to you for your glory, as a memorial of the wonderful things you have already done, and for whatever you plan to do in the future, through this ordeal.
>
> You have taken what the enemy meant for evil, and you have made it good. You still see me as whole and beautiful. You do not look away from the part of my body that is now different, but you love that part just as you did before.

As I prayed, a strange thing happened. I felt that God was anointing my scarred chest with oil. He seemed to be demonstrating to me that he was setting apart my physical loss for his purposes.

It was a holy moment. And though I still occasionally feel sad that I had to lose my breast, I would never trade that moment for the sake of having my breast back.

I don't believe that the comfort I received from God would have been as deep and as longlasting if I hadn't been completely honest with myself and with him about how truly awful I felt. The Psalms are full of examples of God's comfort permeating the heart of the psalmist, who had faced his sorrow and had cried out to God. The author of Psalm 116 writes about God answering him in the midst of his anguish:

I was overcome by trouble and sorrow.
Then I called on the name of the LORD:
"O LORD, save me!"

The LORD is gracious and righteous;
  our God is full of compassion. . . .
When I was in great need, he saved me. . . .

For you, O LORD, have delivered my soul from death,
  my eyes from tears . . .
That I may walk before the LORD
  in the land of the living. (vv. 3-6, 8-9)

There is no evidence that the psalmist shoved his grief aside. Nor did he blame himself for not being "over it" yet or for not being "spiritual" enough to smile and say to all his friends, "I'm fine, thanks." He acknowledged his grief, identified its causes, allowed himself to feel the depths of his sorrow and cried out to God, believing that God would answer him.

Sometimes after we think our grieving has ended, something triggers the grief again. When this happens, we need to pay attention, because our hearts are letting us know that we still have more grieving to do. Often these unexpected situations are opportunities that God has arranged, in which he plans to bring us some further and perhaps final healing. Gerry, for example, remembers watching the televised funeral of Jacqueline Onassis, who had died of cancer. It was a bright, sunny morning, and Gerry found herself sobbing.

To this day I don't know whether I was weeping for her or for myself. But I thought, *I don't care what this is about. I'm going to cry until I don't want to cry any more.* I felt later that it could have been a final grieving for my own experience—that this event in the news had brought about, in a way that other things might never have, the realization that I could identify with her, in leaving her children and so on. My response surprised me a lot, but it was a release for me to cry.

Our grief may not vanish entirely but may lessen in intensity over time. Joan had grieved over losing her breast even before she had her mastectomy, so afterward she was surprised at how long her grieving process still took. "I remember thinking, *Oh, I'm done with it,* but then it would erupt again," she says, "and I would start grieving about it again." Even now, several years later, she occasionally still feels some sorrow over losing her breast. However, Joan's grief has lost most of its depth—so that it's more on the level of "Yeah, it would be nice to have two breasts," she says—and it lasts only a few moments.

Our grief over the specific aspects of our experience with breast cancer can take many forms. And our grief can be short-lived, or it can come and go over a long time. But however complex our grief is, however extended it is, however deep it is, God wants to comfort us and heal our grieving hearts. The apostle Paul says that God is "the Father of compassion and the God of all comfort, who comforts us in all our troubles" (2 Cor 1:3-4). God promises to comfort us in every detail of our grief, whether it's over losing a breast, losing the choice of wearing certain kinds of clothes or losing our lifelong dreams. All we need to do is to be honest with ourselves and with God about our grief and invite him to comfort us.

# 11

## READJUSTING TO NORMAL LIFE

Every aspect of her life was going well for Joan until she found out she had breast cancer. As she became immersed in the onslaught of emotions after her diagnosis and throughout her treatments, she grieved over the loss of her life as she had known it. Although she was able to continue running her hairstyling business, she had to cut back on the number of clients she saw so that she could schedule time for a nap each day. And she didn't have the advantage of paid sick days when she had to miss work after her chemotherapy treatments. In addition, the lives of her husband and children were fiercely shaken because she was less available to them.

Joan had no guarantee that her life would ever be the same again, and she had to determine what *normal* would now mean for her—how many of her clients she would have the strength to see in a day, how much rest she would need, what church activities she may need to give up and whether or not she and her family could take the vacation they had planned.

Not until five months after Joan had finished chemotherapy—about a year after her diagnosis—did she feel entirely like herself again.

Finally she was able to skip her afternoon naps and start seeing more clients each week. She was happy to have her *"new* normal life" back.

But one year later Joan's worst fear about breast cancer was realized: it came back. Suddenly she had to define *normal* all over again, knowing that what had worked before might not work the second time around.

Redefining *normal* has been a continual process for Joan. With each recurrence and then with each recovery period, she has had to make new decisions about what is normal for *her.*

If we're fortunate, we've had to redefine *normal* only once—although we may have made several attempts at redefining it, according to our physical and emotional ups and downs. But no matter how many times we need to redefine it, we're better off if we can identify our physical and emotional limits, test them occasionally and become content to live with our new definitions of *normal* for as long as necessary.

### Longing for Normality

A mistake that many of us make when we're breast cancer novices is that of rushing back into all of our prediagnosis activities. We hate being sick, and we hate for others to think of us as sick. Eager to return to life as healthy, fully functioning individuals, we may become impatient with the slow pace that our bodies require for recovery, and so we plunge back into our routines too soon. Others of us, however, have no regrets about trying to return to a normal routine at the first moment of inspiration, even in a semirecovered condition. For every woman, it's different.

I wasn't very patient with my own body. I have to *move.* I love to dance, using every muscle and every joint as I leap and jump and play with new rhythms and new ways of sculpting the air. Concerned about whether I would regain my full range of movement following surgery, I couldn't wait to find out. So one morning just two weeks after my mastectomy, I selected some lively music, put it into the CD player, turned the volume way up and did some vigorous dance movements across the living room floor for twenty minutes—taking care, of course, not to flail my left arm, which was still sore.

It was gratifying to describe this accomplishment later to my friends who would call and ask how I was feeling. Wanting to hear friends exclaim about how well I was doing had perhaps been part of my motivation for resuming physical activities so soon. More to the point, though, I wanted to prove to *myself* that my recovery would be quick and that the time lost from my daily routine would be short. Fortunately, I didn't suffer any physical repercussions from my zealousness that day or any other day, so I don't regret indulging myself. But I knew I was pushing the limits. If I had it to do over (and I hope I never do), I might wait a few more days.

Margo realized that she too had been a bit eager in her efforts to recover from surgery. As an elder in her church, she served communion, as scheduled, the Sunday after her mastectomy. "I think I was trying to make everything normal—just the same as it always was," she says, "and prove to myself that I could do it. But I remember afterward thinking, *That was so foolish; I can't believe I did that.*"

Serving communion and dancing were conservative activities compared with what Elena did following her mastectomy. She stunned her husband by announcing on their way out of the hospital, "I want to go camping." Drainage tubes still hanging from her incision, she gathered together some camping supplies as soon as she got home from the hospital, and amid her husband's protests, they left the next day. "We went camping, and I forgot about my breast," she says. "I was a little bit weak. But I saw the trees, and I saw the squirrels in the trees, and I thought, *Ah! It's so beautiful! I have so much freedom here. This is life!*"

Whether or not Elena, Margo and I made the right decisions about our activities is beside the point; the real issue is that all of us who have had breast cancer have shared a deep longing to return to life as it had been before—and the sooner the better.

Occasionally I hear a woman who has breast cancer say that she feels guilty for longing to return to normal and that she wants to become content with her current physical condition, which she cannot control. Her struggle is understandable. The apostle Paul says, "I have learned the secret of being content in any and every situation" (Phil 4:12). He then tells us that secret: "I can do everything through him who gives me strength" (v. 13). Does this mean that the yearning to return to normal is wrong? How do we become content when our circumstances are constantly changing? What does it mean to "do everything through him who gives me strength" when we're recovering from breast cancer and we can plan our lives only one week at a time, or perhaps just a few hours at a time? We may be asking ourselves, *Will I have as much strength and alertness tomorrow as I have today? Will I be able to work full-time again soon? Will I ever be able to resume all the normal activities that I enjoyed doing before I had cancer?* And *Is God displeased that I have this terrible longing to go back to my normal routine?* So how do we resolve this tension between longing to return to normal and becoming content with our present circumstances?

As we spend time with God—asking him questions, thanking him for his good gifts and receiving his love for us—we get to know him better. And as we get to know him better, his desires become our desires. "Delight yourself in the LORD and he will give you the desires of your heart," says the psalmist (Ps 37:4). God does not tell us to make sure that our desires are acceptable to him before we come to him; he tells us simply to come to him, believing that Jesus, through his death and resurrection, has made our relationship with God possible, and asking with thankful hearts for what we want (Phil 4:6-7).

God invites us to bring every longing of our hearts to him—our longing to be fully available to our families and friends and church communities, our longing to not be cooped up at home, our longing to dance or swim or play tennis, our longing to be free of the pain or discomfort resulting from cancer or from our treatments, our longing to feel normal again. These are healthy things to ask God for. They represent life, and God, who is the source of all life, wants us to choose life. We can freely ask him to fill our longings, confident that either he'll give them to us or he'll help us find contentment without them.

## Becoming Content

To become content in every situation, as the apostle Paul was able to do by receiving strength from Christ, sometimes means that we need to lower our expectations of ourselves. Gerry did that during her five weeks of radiation treatments. Disappointed that she wouldn't be able to take her annual summertime trips to see family members, she consoled herself by improving the appearance and comfort of the place where she would spend much of her summer—her front porch.

One day when she felt strong enough to run errands with her husband, Howard, she found some wicker furniture that exactly matched the color of their house. They bought it and placed it on their porch, and Gerry used it regularly to entertain friends or to sit with Howard on warm evenings.

For the many years that I've known Gerry she has grown roses along the path from the sidewalk to her front steps. There, on familiar territory, some pleasant surprises awaited her that summer.

> I couldn't walk any farther than the driveway and the sidewalk; I was on a very short tether at that time. But as I would go out and talk to my roses and water them, I found that people walking by would stop. They didn't know I'd had surgery, but we would visit about roses. Some of those people I never saw again, but it delighted me to find that kind of relationship almost at my front door.

Gerry felt that the passers-by she met from her vacation spot were gifts from God that helped her to become content. She tells of a man who stopped to talk with her one morning when she greeted him.

> He was about forty and was wearing a backpack, and I said, "You look like you're going to school." And he was. I think I told him I'd had surgery, and he told me he'd had brain surgery or something. But here he was, going forward into some new experience for himself. That encouraged me a lot. I might not have known it if I hadn't said hello to him. And that was right out in my front yard.

When we look for ways that God wants to meet us, he sometimes surprises us with special gifts.

### Helping a Woman to Feel Normal

Those who want to help us readjust to our normal routines can best do so by interacting with us as if we were completely healthy. This doesn't mean ignoring our current or recent experience of breast cancer; we still want others to be interested in how we're doing, pray for us and give us practical help if we need it. But we also don't want to be looked at as different or as less capable than we were before we had breast cancer.

After starting yet another series of chemotherapy for a recurrence of her breast cancer, Joan was dismayed one day to find out that her name had been removed from the list of volunteers who took turns leading worship and serving refreshments for one of her Bible study groups. She felt hurt that the others had assumed, without asking her, that she would not want to continue doing such tasks. To her, it was as if they were no longer *permitting* her to do those things. However, when someone from another women's group that Joan belonged to invited Joan to begin serving on a committee, Joan responded, "You don't know how much this means to me—the fact that you've asked me. This shows that you still see me as a useful human being." Joan didn't decide right then whether or not to accept the invitation, but she was pleased to be given the choice. "I've got to keep living, and I've got to be doing these things myself," she explains. "Don't take those things from me."

Whether we're still undergoing treatment or we've completed treatment, we don't want our lives to stop. We need to have other things to think about besides our disease and how our lives have been shaken by it. Taking on a few responsibilities, if we have the strength, can help us to feel not only that we're still human and still useful but also that there's still some semblance of normality in our lives.

Our family members need to be included in normal activities as much as we need to be. Joan's husband, George, was invited to serve as an elder of their church. When George told the news to Greg, a friend and fellow leader in the church, Greg looked aghast and said, "But I told them not to ask you. That makes me mad!" He apparently was concerned that George would feel offended by being asked to take on new responsibilities while his wife was fighting breast cancer.

"But I said yes," George said to Greg.

Greg stared at George incredulously and then threw up his hands. "OK, I give up," he said.

What Greg didn't understand was that George needed to feel like he had a fairly normal life, even though it had been vigorously shaken by his wife's breast cancer. We can only guess what other people will want or not want when they're in a crisis, and trying to guess may hurt them. Although they themselves may not know what they want, they appreciate being given a choice. We're unlikely to offend them if we say something like what the church leaders had told George when they invited him to be an elder: "We know you've got a lot going on in your life right now, but we just want to ask you. And if you say yes and it becomes too much and you need to take a leave of absence, it's no problem." An invitation of that sort can help the woman who has breast cancer or her husband or child feel like a normal person, and feel included and valued, even if the responsibility being offered would be too difficult to accept.

Whereas we might be excluded from normal activities when we're recovering from breast cancer, we might also experience the opposite: being expected to participate in normal activities when we can't. Viola looked fairly normal following her chemotherapy, radiation, high-dose chemo and stem-cell transplant, even though she had been sick and exhausted for a long time. People often told her that if they hadn't known otherwise, they never would have guessed what she had been through. And some of them at times asked her to participate in activities, forgetting that she might still feel exhausted or that she sometimes had to isolate herself because of her very low white-blood-cell count and weakened immune system.

> The only time I had a problem when asked to help in a way I couldn't was at a church I was attending. That was probably the hardest thing for me to deal with; I don't say no easily. There was an obvious rebuff when the person turned their back and said, "Just never mind." It took a while before I could really feel that the problem was not with me.

Again, the solution seems to lie in giving us a choice of saying yes or no—a genuine choice, not layered with overtones of expectations, like the choice that Viola was given.

Supporting someone who is trying to feel normal can at times be awkward and difficult. It can be even more awkward and difficult if that person is not expected to survive. Margaret has some suggestions that can apply equally to those of us who are recovering:

> Everyone seems to look at me as something unique now, someone set apart, different. And what I need is to feel normal; the joy I find in the dailyness of life is real important. To do normal things with others is a real joy—to have them to dinner, to just sit and have a cup of tea, to help

them wash dishes, all of the normal things. It makes me feel like I'm not unique. It's a small thing, but it's a part of what separates those who have been a support to me and those who have not. We don't have to sit and talk about my disease; I don't have to be "sick." We can talk about life—just anything, just normal things. We can talk about the Lord. It's a relief to me. It keeps me focused on the healthy things of life.

What we all need is to feel normal. Whether we're still fighting cancer or we're trying to make peace with the memories of fighting cancer, we need, as much as possible, to be allowed to do the daily routine tasks that we would do if we were completely healthy. Whether we survive two more months or forty more years, we need to *live*. We can go to the Author of life and ask him to fill all our longings and to help us feel normal again. He is pleased when we choose life.

---

While we redefine *normal* by adapting to our circumstances, we can also do certain things to help ourselves feel normal. The ideas mentioned here may be obvious to you, or you may have already created your own list. But sometimes when we've been ill we need to be reminded of our options.

■ When you feel well enough to go out, go out. Invite a friend or family member to go with you. Go shopping. Go to a movie. Go someplace where you can watch the world around you.

■ When the weather is pleasant, go to a park, find a bench to sit on (or take a mat and pillow with you if you're more comfortable lying down) and enjoy the action. Watch the children playing. Watch the dogs chasing after balls. Watch the clouds forming overhead. Listen to the birds singing, the squirrels scampering through the trees and the ducks quacking. Take a chance and greet someone who has a friendly face.

■ On days that you don't feel well enough to leave home, go outside for a few minutes to see what's growing, to watch the clouds, to get some sunshine or to catch some snowflakes or raindrops on your tongue.

■ Invite a friend to meet you for lunch. Talk about your cancer experience, but talk about other topics as well. And if your friend seems to feel awkward, be patient with her. Tell her how you feel about your cancer experience and about how much or how little you want to talk about it. Consider telling her also how she can best help you during this readjustment phase (for suggestions, see Appendix C).

■ If you become discouraged about your slow recovery and all the things you still can't do, make a list of the things you *can* do that you enjoy, and do them often. Keep the list handy in case you become discouraged again.

■ Think of something new you'd like to try that's within your current capabilities—drawing, gardening, writing, origami, stock market speculation, astronomy or a computer program.

■ Find out who in your church or among your friends or coworkers is sick or has needs similar to the needs that you had during your cancer treatment. Write them notes to let them know that you're thinking of them and praying for them.

■ Buy a telephone that has more speed-dial buttons than your old one. Program it with phone numbers of friends whom you've been wanting to get to know better, and start calling them more often.

■ Learn to program your VCR. Then offer to record special shows for friends and neighbors who still can't program theirs.

# 12

## SEEING
## OURSELVES IN
## NEW WAYS

One of the ironies of having breast cancer is that throughout our entire treatment phase we can hardly wait until we've recovered. Lying across our beds in a half-stupor, we may fantasize about the luxury of putting on our pantyhose and returning to a forty-hour work week or planning our children's next birthday party. Never before have board meetings, carpool responsibilities and closet reorganizing sounded so good, and we promise ourselves we'll never take them for granted again. Yet, when our treatments are over and we're finally feeling more or less ourselves, we may be disappointed. Although easing back into our routines may hold some pleasure for us, it feels different somehow.

Maybe nothing around us has changed much. But then we realize that *we* are different. Breast cancer has left a mark on us that goes way beyond scars and a disrupted schedule. As we look inward at ourselves, we may recognize a lingering fear that our cancer will return and will get us next time. At the same time, we may discover a new sense of urgency about setting new priorities and achieving certain goals. We may value each day a little more. And we may realize that God has helped us to grow in some extraordinary ways.

### Facing Lingering Fears

Even if our treatments are far behind us, we may find that breast cancer has left us with a fear or an anxiety that stalks us and pounces on us unexpectedly. It might subtly creep up into our throats when we're anticipating our annual mammogram or when we feel an unfamiliar pain. Or it might kick us in the stomach when we find out that someone else we know has been diagnosed with cancer, especially if it's a recurrence. "I will never be free of the knowledge that someday it could hit again," says Rachel. Although she was treated for colon cancer in 1994, she has had no recurrences of her breast cancer. But she has lingering fears.

The fear of recurrence can be inhibiting. "I still feel anxious when I go for my oncology checkups," says Judy. "I miss the carefreeness of just being healthy," says Connie, "and I think of death more often." And Gerry says that even now, several years after her treatments, she gets "very nervous and jumpy" when she returns for her annual checkup. "I still get the 'what-ifs' in the night and in the darker moments," she says.

Getting regular checkups offers us a mixed bag of anxiety and relief. While we may feel anxious about what the doctor will say, we're relieved when we hear good news. "As I got closer to an appointment with the oncologist, probably the feelings would erupt more," says Joan, describing the period of time before her first recurrence. "And after seeing him and being told, 'You're fine,' I would leave and feel good again, and that would recharge me for a long time—that length of time before my next visit."

There are ways that we can minimize our fears, even if we can't eradicate them. After years of undergoing annual mammograms that have turned out fine, I still dread each autumn, when it's time to schedule another one. This may sound paranoid, but when I show up for the appointment, I always ask the technologist to write a note to the radiologist, requesting that the mammogram report be immediately faxed to my primary-care doctor. And because my doctor works part-time, I always schedule my mammogram for one day prior to a day that she plans to be in her office. That way, I can get the results just one day later. As relatively easy as my own experience with breast cancer was, I don't want to ever have to go through it again. Nor do I want to wait a week to find out if I'll have to. So I take those practical steps to deal with my own lingering fear.

Another lingering fear can directly result from completing our treatments. Undergoing regular treatments for our cancer helps us to feel that we're doing everything possible to actively fight the cancer; the end of the treatments, conversely, can make us feel vulnerable again. Nancy says she went through a grieving period over the completion of her treatments, because she was no longer doing something to fight her cancer. And Jane, after finishing chemotherapy, remembers thinking, *Well, it better have worked. Because if there's just one more little cell that needed to be killed off.* . . . Jane feels somewhat reassured by the tamoxifen that she's now taking, but she anticipates that when it's time for her to stop the tamoxifen, she'll have "another one of those feelings."

Other common lingering fears include the fear of having to undergo treatment once more and to again suffer side effects such as nausea, pain and fatigue. We may also fear the hardship of having our lives disrupted again by cancer. The disruption often goes beyond inconvenience; we can't afford the time away from work, or we're the only available caregivers to our aging parents, or we have children at home who need our undistracted attention.

No matter what prompts our fear or what forms the fear takes, the basic, underlying fear is usually the same: that the cancer will come back, and when it does, we'll die. Margaret got a call from a woman she had never met, who was in Margaret's church and had heard about Margaret's recurrence of breast cancer, which had metastasized. The caller—we'll call her Carol—was fighting breast cancer herself and had just completed chemotherapy treatments. On the day that she called Margaret, Carol was about to go to her first recall visit to her oncologist, an event that has made many breast cancer patients feel like prisoners going before a parole board, hoping to be told "You're free."

Carol's stated purpose in the call was to offer her support to Margaret. "I'll be praying for you, and I want to do whatever I can to help you," she said enthusiastically. However, as Carol's own story unfolded, Margaret began to hear between Carol's words an undercurrent of fear. Margaret decided to be blunt: "Are you imagining that what's happening to me is going to happen to *you* someday?" she asked.

A silence passed between them for a moment, and then Carol began to cry. "Yeah. It's been eating me up all day. I just can't get past the idea that it's going to come back and get me."

Margaret gently reminded Carol that God knows exactly what each person needs. "Don't presume that you're going to have a recurrence of breast cancer just because *I* have," she added. "That isn't right. God is still in control."

Carol's fear is common and completely normal. We don't displease God by being afraid. But he wants to replace our fears with the confidence that he loves us, that he is always with us and that nothing is beyond his control. That confidence may be based on an experience of God's comforting presence in the midst of cancer, as well as on his promises to us in the Bible. Having experienced his presence after our first diagnosis, we can be confident that God would be with us during a recurrence, if we were to have one.

Nancy, who was first diagnosed in 1990 and had a recurrence about five years later, says she's "working on" that confidence.

> This is one place where the statistics and my faith clash. I believe that God can and does heal, regardless of what medical wisdom and statistics say. I also believe that the statistics continue to require attention, because there is some measure of truth to them. Reconciling God's plan for me as he sees it, God's plan for me as I would like it to be and cancer statistics is a major trapeze act for me. Having had one recurrence, should I expect another?
>
> But I'm beginning to understand what it means to abide in Christ. The waiting and wondering about recurrence hangs very heavy. It seems that abiding in Christ is the antidote to the fears. I need to learn to enjoy today and not worry about tomorrow or next year or twenty years from now. That is a continuing process. I need to affirm my faith in a loving Father who has everything under control, who never errs, who is with me "to the end."

Although Janaha experienced breast cancer indirectly, having lost her mother to the disease, she often fears getting cancer the first time. But she too relies on God to comfort her in her fears.

> Sometimes it really scares me, because *I don't want to get cancer,* and I don't want to have children if I have to go through that; I know how it affected *me.* But having watched my mother persevere to the end, if I were to get sick, I'd feel equipped, in some way, to handle the situation and not feel ignorant. So I guess there's a part of me that thinks, *If I were to get sick, then I'm going to be OK, regardless.* Because there's this faith that God is going to make it right. And that keeps me strong.

This confidence does not happen to us suddenly, in most cases. It usually develops over time, as we continue to reflect on our experiences of God's presence during cancer and as we present every fear and every anxiety to him.

### Recognizing Personal Growth

I don't believe that God's plan in allowing me to have breast cancer was simply to make me a better person. I still wince every time someone responds to my personal story with, "Oh, so for you it was a character-building experience." Sure, it was. So is looking for a parking place in downtown San Francisco during rush hour when it's pouring rain and I have a headache and I'm almost late for an appointment. For many of us, having breast cancer did much more than build character. It was a landmark time in our lives when God proved himself to us—proved his love, his goodness and his faithfulness—in ways that we had never experienced before. It was a time in which he gave us the gift of discovering more of who we are and who he is.

Some of us have learned through our experience how crucial it is to face our feelings. Sarah believes that in other crises she hasn't faced her feelings as squarely as she has with her breast cancer. "I haven't coped with them in the right way, and there have been repercussions later on. But I do feel, at last, that my relationship with God has deepened and is strengthened."

Nancy, who had a recurrence, regrets that she didn't face her fears right away, after either diagnosis.

I had mild feelings that I should keep a journal at the outset of the second go-'round. But I couldn't, I think mainly because I was unwilling to face my fears and my lack of faith. Somehow putting them down in pen and ink made them more cast in concrete. I come from a practiced line of "ostriches." The modeling was, *If I don't acknowledge this situation, these feelings, they are not so real.* It's not easy to break that mindset. If I could have written them down, they probably would have taken on reasonable proportions and I could have systematically dealt with them. As it was, they just flew around in my mind and made trouble for me.

Whether we faced our feelings right after our diagnosis or not until much later, it's never too late to benefit in some way from our cancer experience. Jane, the college dean and mother of two, sees several ways that her cancer experience has caused her to grow. First, she feels confident that she'll be able to handle any future crises in her life with grace and dignity—at least any crisis that happens mainly to her. (Understandably, she's less confident about how she would handle a crisis involving her children.) Second, she is more willing now to accept help from others when she needs it, for both their benefit and hers. And third, she believes that God is answering one of the questions she had asked him—What should I be learning from this?—by giving her a yearning for his rest and peace in the midst of a very busy life. She does become discouraged at times, however, and asks herself, *Why can't you get your life in a little bit more order?* "I work hard," she says, "and I have high expectations for myself as a mother as well as for my work at the college."

But Jane recognizes how God has used her cancer to change her attitude about her hectic pace. "I know that the cancer could come back and that I could die. I don't think there's the same innocence. But maybe the newly sobered Jane is more willing to allow God to do what he needs to do in my life and not to hold on to it as tightly."

Bonita, like Jane, is concerned about the stresses in her life. She recognizes how God has used her cancer experience to help her reevaluate her priorities in trying to balance her work with the probation department program and her dedication to her family.

I was on a cycle of being supermom, superwoman, superperson at work, and doing it all, and there was no end to it. And I think God kind of took control of that. It slowed me down; it put things into perspective. On your job, you think, *If I don't do it, it won't get done,* but if you're off on sick leave, you find out things *do* get done, things do go on. And it helps you to say, "OK, my family is more important than the job, because I'm the mama here, and they only have one mother, whereas at work they can always put somebody else in my position."

Allowing God to change us through our breast cancer experience— that is, presenting ourselves to him and inviting him to change us—is more important to God than how hard we work to become changed. In fact, the Bible says that a changed heart is God's responsibility, whereas our responsibility is to open our hearts to him and to let him guide us and empower us to make necessary changes. Paul assures us that "he who began a good work in you will carry it on to completion" (Phil 1:6) and that God's power is "made perfect in weakness" (2 Cor 12:9). Bonita has experienced God's power in her own weakness:

I see that I'm a better person for what I've gone through—that in acknowledging my weakness, I'm also acknowledging God's strength. Although I probably thought it and said it and certainly was taught it my whole life—that God is in control and he determines how long we live—it never struck home as real as it did when I was faced with my own mortality at age thirty-six, when everything was going really well in my life.

Margaret, who retired at age forty-nine from her career as a bed-and-breakfast innkeeper, learned from having breast cancer that she was "infinitely weaker" than she had thought she was. But she's careful to point out how that self-perception is not the same as low self-esteem:

The difference is, where is the credit, who gets the glory? I've been blessed in terms of the abilities that God has given me, and I've accomplished many of my goals in this life. But there were times that I misused those gifts, particularly in my business. I took the credit for them more often than not. I got real big-headed; I was a hot shot. But the truth is that those gifts are from God. Relative to self-esteem, the good that is in me is a gift from him. Whatever good I have accomplished in this life is an act of his grace. And my character is enriched when I give the glory to God. So I like it better this way. There's less stress involved, because I don't have an image to protect. And I think God can be honored much better, because I recognize that I'm weak.

Although recognizing our weakness in light of God's strength is a good position to be in, God can strengthen us in areas in which we need to be strong. Following a painful conversation with her daughter one day, in which they worked through some difficulties in their relationship, Gerry recognized how God had strengthened her.

> My daughter said, "Wow! You're *strong*. You stayed with me all through that conversation." And I said, "Well, I've faced cancer." In hearing myself say that, I realized that I had faced down my fears and come through an awesome and traumatic experience. It *did* make me stronger and more confident in myself and more willing to be real. Her observation was very helpful to me, so that now I pray with a lot more confidence. I *know* God is hearing me; I *know* he's there. I question sometimes what I ought to be praying *for* myself, but it's always, "What would you have of me? What is your purpose for me now, and how can I work with you toward your goal for me?" Because I think there are going to be new dreams and new ambitions and maybe new energies. I can pray with strength and conviction now in a way that I never did before.

One of our greatest areas of potential growth when we've had breast cancer is our capacity to receive love both from God and from others. Gerry discovered not only how strong she had become but also how much she is loved. She hadn't before experienced "that deep, deep knowledge of God's love," she says, but through the many people who demonstrated love to her, she now sees herself "more deeply as a person of great worth in God's eyes." Sarah, who had always struggled with low self-esteem, also says that her breast cancer experience has made her much more aware of God's love for her. And many of the women I interviewed say that their increased awareness of God's love has given them more compassion for others, not only for people who have cancer but for anyone who is suffering.

Some of those women have found that God is using them in new ways to share his love and compassion with others. Viola, who has suffered some severe physical injuries as well as several recurrences of cancer, is one example:

I now see that God has taken me through all of the cancers and injuries because he wants me to be ready, full-time, to be there for others who are confronted with cancer or other life-threatening illnesses. When I was feeling better, I took on the personality of Iris the Clown and worked with our local hospice. This was a very special way to share with others what God has done for me, and it was wonderful to bring a smile to the faces of the patients and their families. The great thing about Iris and patients is that they will tell her things they won't even tell their nurse, because Iris is nonthreatening. This has been a great open door that came directly from my original cancer.

Expressing God's love and compassion to others is a natural outgrowth of allowing God to change our values. Margaret has seen the difference that her changed values have made in her own life, especially in how she relates to others:

My priorities are much clearer. I'm not distracted by the things of the world, because I don't need them; they're irrelevant. What's important are people. And God. And how I can interact between the two and be a catalyst for change in people's lives toward God. That's my mission. I have a mission, and I'm zealous about it; I'm *jealous* about it. I'm real careful on one issue, though: it's his agenda; it isn't mine. My whole life I've had my own agenda of what was important and what I wanted to accomplish. In the last year, I have learned to stop it and to rest in the Lord and wait on him and let him bring to me what he wants me to do. So I'm not going out seeking anything; I'm waiting for him to bring the opportunities to me. And he's doing that.

Judy says she is no longer the workaholic that she was before she was diagnosed.

Breast cancer changed my view of my life. I now see it as a valuable and fragile gift from God. I now strive to emphasize things of eternal value: spending time with the Lord, writing a devotional book, mentoring college/career women and using the gifts God has given me. I value my small measure of physical health by taking better care of myself through nutrition, rest and exercise, and I value family members by keeping in contact by phone and letters and by making more trips to visit them.

Having breast cancer goes way beyond character building. When we allow God to intervene in our experience with breast cancer, our perspectives change, our values change and we grow in our understanding of ourselves and of God.

### Discovering a New Sense of Urgency

Breast cancer reminds us that we don't know how much time we'll have on earth. And that reminder is so powerful that we're never quite the same afterward. We don't look at ourselves in the same ways, which means that we don't look at others in the same ways or at our resources, especially our time, in the same ways.

Gerry finds that the fear of a recurrence of her cancer has given her a new sense of urgency. "I have to get things done," she says, "because I know I'm vulnerable." When she was receiving cancer treatment, she realized how desperately she wanted to fulfill some of her longtime dreams, so now she's working toward those goals. One of her dreams is to write about her family's history and present it to her children and grandchildren. For years Gerry has researched her family's history, and now, to make the writing process easier, she is learning how to use a computer, with help from her husband, a semiretired engineer.

John, whose first wife—my friend Karen—died of breast cancer, is glad that he and Karen never put off vacations or other meaningful activities, even before Karen became ill. Sixteen years later, her illness and death still remind him not to put off the important things. "You can't live your life on interpersonal credit, like you're going to pull off all these wonderful things in some rosy, distant time when you have time to get to them," John says. "You've got to do them when you can, and not expect that you'll have another chance."

While recognizing a new sense of urgency within ourselves can help us choose how to spend our time, it can sometimes cause internal conflicts. Connie, for example, often has thoughts like, *Maybe I should get all my pictures into the picture book* and *Maybe I'd better write down all the things that I want my grandchildren to know about me and my walk with God.* Connie also struggles, as many of us do, with how to communicate with others about what God has done in her life.

Margo's experience with cancer reminded her that the days are short and that every day is valuable. That sense of urgency, for her, sometimes takes the form of impatience. "I feel impatient with easy-answer kinds of people—especially church people," she says. "Easy answers always troubled me. Now they don't just trouble me; they make me crazy. I can't listen to them."

Margaret explains that impatience:

> I think that God gives you special grace to get through a crisis—people are praying, they're sending cards, they're bringing food, they're paying attention to you, and there's all this action. And then it kind of dwindles. You're not in treatment any more, you look normal, your hair has grown back, you're fitting back into the routine of things. But you're not the same. There are parts of you that are very different, and some of the things that used to work don't work any more. Not only your body but your coping mechanisms. Somehow, your perspective is different. You *have* faced your own mortality, and there is almost an impatience with those who haven't done that yet.

Believing that she needs to spend her remaining months focused on God, Margaret cites Moses' prayer, "Teach us to number our days aright, that we may gain a heart of wisdom" (Ps 90:12). To Margaret, that means submitting our minds to God, asking him to help us see our lives from his perspective. "All of our time is short here on earth," she says, "and compared to eternity, we have such a brief time to gain wisdom."

Because some of our values have changed, we may even talk differently. Frieda recalls overhearing a skirmish among two coworkers who were "going ballistic over some stupid little thing." One of them then walked away, sneering over her shoulder to the other one, "Get a life!" Frieda reflected on that incident the next day as she drove to work.

> I thought, *It's way deeper than that—about whether somebody doesn't cross their t or dot their i. It's like, instead of saying, "Get a life!" you say, "Get a death!"* So when I got to work I told Liz about that—she's a coworker who had cancer before I did—and she said, "That's it. Things that we hear people stressing about around here are so trivial when you're faced with life and death." So that was our little private saying: "Get a death!"

The new sense of urgency we often experience after having breast cancer can be a useful and valuable tool. It can help us to see ourselves differently, to use our time more efficiently and to realize how thoroughly dependent we are on God for who we are and who we're becoming.

## Living One Day at a Time

As students in the school of cancer, we've learned the importance of living one day at a time. When we live one day at a time, we enjoy God's daily gifts to us on a deeper level and we become less afraid of the future.

Margaret was surprised that after her cancer had advanced, she felt more "earthly minded" rather than "spiritually minded." She adopted an I-want-it-now attitude: "I was no longer willing to delay gratification," she says. "I guess I had come face to face with my own mortality, and I said, 'Well, I'm not going to wait for that vacation' or for that new carpet or whatever it was I wanted." Troubled by that attitude, she soon saw how living one day at a time could help her:

> I learned what it meant to really, really enjoy what life had to offer that day. Every day that I wake up feeling good I praise God. I don't have a clue about what tomorrow will bring, and it doesn't matter. Today I feel good, I have energy, I'm interested in life, I can drive my car, and that's enough. To make the most of *today* is enough.

Margaret also sees living one day at a time as an opportunity for God to use us in other people's lives:

> It's delicious to fill a day with good things and to be aware that that's what you're doing. I love the word *effective*—to make today effective, for Christ and for me, for my family, for people I love. It puts a whole new twist on everything that I do; it makes it matter. And I can have *fun* that way. I don't have to be morbid, and I don't have to sit around and suck my thumb. I can thoroughly enjoy whatever is happening at the moment, because the moment is where I am.

Eighteen years after having breast cancer and more recently having her perspective underscored by her husband's serious health problems, Rachel sees living one day at a time as a long-term benefit. "God has used all these medical problems to teach Robert and me to live one day at a time," she says. "If you want to live life as well as possible, you need to live each day and feel good about it and be aware that we have *today*—no promises for tomorrow."

Living one day at a time means enjoying and being grateful for the ordinary things that today is filled with: the smell of fresh coffee, the softness of cotton clothing, the voice of a friend on the phone, the beauty of a child's face. It means to savor each moment that we receive such gifts.

Savoring the moment is not something I learned by having breast cancer. It's a concept I learned as a child, when I realized that I had only a few more days to enjoy the texture of grass under my bare feet before I would have to start school again. But having breast cancer added a new dimension to that concept: I'm thankful to God for every blade of that grass. My brush with mortality has made me feel that waking up to each new day is like getting an extension on the deadline for a term paper when I was in college. Or celebrating my birthday with people I love. Or going on a long-awaited vacation. Or coming home to John when I've been traveling alone. Ordinary tasks—paying bills, standing in line at the post office, vacuuming the same spider webs from the upper corners of my living room that I'm sure I vacuumed two weeks ago—become privileges instead of drudgery.

I treasure each moment that I hear the voices of my two young nieces, Heather and Lauren, on the phone; the next time I see them, they'll be a little more grown up than they are today. In the springtime I always breathe deeply as I walk by the freesias planted in our front yard, because they'll be dried up in a few weeks. And I don't leave my house without embracing John—or let him leave without embracing me—because I never know if it will be my last chance to feel his cheek pressed against mine. I know that life is as fragile as a freesia blossom and as transient as childhood.

No, I don't dwell on morbid thoughts; I don't live in fear that I'm going to suddenly die and lose all the treasures of life that I cling to. Rather, I live in gratitude to God that I'm here for another moment, another day. Today is a gift from him, crammed with other gifts: the taste of hot pizza with spicy tomato sauce and lots of garlic (hold the cheese), the laughter of children playing at a daycare center over the fence from our house, a friend's reassuring arm around my shoulder—

even a virtual gesture of affection through an e-mail message. God does not owe me any of these things. But he is a generous God who delights in giving good gifts to his children, and I gladly receive whatever he chooses to give me today.

# 13

## SEEING DEATH
## IN NEW
## WAYS

Cancer equals death. That's how many of the women I talked with said they felt about cancer before they were diagnosed and immediately afterward. Most of the people they had ever known who had had cancer had died of it; therefore, they reasoned, they would die too.

As Christians, we believe that Jesus died and was resurrected to set us free from the power of death, and that for us, dying means going home—leaving our earthly bodies behind and having our spirits instantaneously transported into heaven, where we will live forever with God. But no matter how sincerely we may believe these things, death is still a monstrous enemy that we deeply fear and dread. We fear what it might really be like for our spirits to leave our bodies. We fear the pain that we may have to suffer. We dread leaving our children or our grandchildren. We dread the grief and loneliness that all of our loved ones will feel when we die, because we remember how we felt when someone we love died. And we can't get excited about going to heaven when we still have so many plans and goals and dreams to fulfill here on earth.

The Bible shows us that God understands our fear and our dread of

death. Jesus wept on his way to Lazarus's tomb, even though he was
about to raise Lazarus from the dead (Jn 11:35). As Jesus anguished in
prayer over his own death, his sweat "was like drops of blood falling to
the ground" (Lk 22:44). And when King Hezekiah wept bitterly and
cried out to God on his deathbed, God mercifully promised to add
fifteen years to his life (2 Kings 20:1-11).

We have a compassionate God, who knew before we were ever born
when and how we would die. Because he is compassionate, he wants to
take away our fear of death. But even more than that, he wants to help
us see death as he sees it. Whenever we face the possibility, or the
likelihood, of impending death—our own or someone else's—we are
forever changed. But we can be changed in positive ways. If we turn to
God with our fears and our dread, he will give us new, positive ways of
looking at death.

## Facing the Fear of Our Own Death

A hallmark of the Christian life is to believe that "to live is Christ and
to die is gain" (Phil 1:21). Perhaps for years we have genuinely believed
that, but when our lives are threatened by breast cancer we may
suddenly struggle with whether death would be indeed a gain. We may
believe that being in heaven with Jesus is infinitely better than our most
glorious days on earth. But given the choice about being with him now,
we would probably say, "Lord, please let me raise my children," or "I
want to see my grandchildren," or "My life is finally starting to impact
other people," or "My husband needs me," or "I haven't yet fulfilled
my lifelong dream." Rachel struggled with that dilemma for nearly a
year. "As I got away from the experience of diagnosis and treatment—as
I felt better and life was feeling more normal—I found myself holding
on to life. I didn't want to let go; I wasn't ready."

Janaha remembers one day when her mother did not feel ready. She
looked at her teenage daughter, began to cry, then grabbed her and
said, "Janaha, I don't want to die. I want to see you get married and
have children." Her mother, who Janaha says had a very nurturing
heart, was grieving over the loss of her dreams. "That stuck with me,"
Janaha says. "I just held her, because I saw her vulnerability."

Janaha did observe, however, that her mother received strength and

comfort from God to face her own death. And she watched as her
mother's supernatural strength overflowed to others.

> People would come to her for prayer and for advice; every person who
> came to our house, she'd minister to. They would pray together, and my
> mom would encourage *anyone.* She actually brought a woman to the
> Lord not even a month before she died. And everyone who came left
> either in tears or completely blessed.

As she saw how her mother received strength from God, Janaha
herself felt strengthened to face her own death someday. "It's not as
scary any more," she says. "I went through a stage in which I was afraid
of getting cancer. I would think, *How could I handle this?* I felt strong,
though—like, *Well, I've watched my mother go through this, and I'd be strong;
I could handle this.* Through the strength of God, I could handle it."

Rachel, who kept "holding on to life," also found comfort and peace
from God after about a year of not being willing to face death. "I have
strong memories," she says, "of that place of my relationship with God
and saying, 'Yeah. It's OK.'"

Bonita had spent a summer praying, "Lord, I want to be closer to
you; I want to know you more." But she soon regretted that prayer.

> I prayed that prayer, and I got cancer. So I've been very hesitant to say
> that again, I must admit. And I've had guilt about that. It's like, "Lord,
> I still want to be close to you, but I don't want you to have to take me
> through that kind of experience again for me to have that relationship
> with you. Let's just do it an easier way."
>
> To me, that's limiting my trust in him. That's me telling the Lord what
> I want. It used to kind of upset me when my father would always pray,
> "Lord, your will be done." I wanted him to say, "Lord, heal her, heal her,
> heal her." I didn't know what his will *was.* I want the Lord's will to be
> done, but I want it to be done so that I can still be here. So in a way, it's
> not wanting to let go of my life completely. But I feel like, even in recent
> months, I've made progress with that.

For Bonita, "recent months" meant nine years after being diagnosed. So the process of letting go of our lives and trusting God can be
ongoing. Bonita's progress became clear to her recently when she
found another lump in her breast. Until she was told that the lump was

benign, she again faced the fear of dying.

> I almost felt like, "Well, Lord, if this is a recurrence and it's time, then I guess that's it." Whereas before, I was always fighting it: *I don't want to die, I don't want to die, I don't want to die.* And this time it almost scared me, like, *Now, why am I feeling a peace about dying? Does that mean I'm going to die?* Because I'd just gotten to the point where I'm more trusting. So it's helped me to see that when it's my time, God will be with me. And I can honestly say that I have less fear now than I did years ago. Now, more than ever, I believe I can have peace with dying. As I've grown older and seen what God can do, I trust his love.

Joan, who has had several recurrences, has found that she too has less fear about dying: "A half a year ago, I couldn't have faced it; I was going nuts with the thought." But now, she says, "people look at me and ask, 'How can you carry on? How do you go from day to day?' God does it *for* me somehow."

No matter how great is our fear of death, no matter how we waver in our faith, God is with us, to relieve our fear and to comfort us with his peace. We can see death as a gain compared with our present lives. We can trust his love for us.

### Facing the Death of a Loved One

When someone we care about dies of breast cancer, how do we as Christians respond in a culture that tends to hide death and those who are dying? And how does God use the experience of someone else's death to strengthen our faith? John, whose first wife, Karen, died of breast cancer in 1981, found that his belief in what the Bible says about eternal life made a big difference in how he grieved over his wife's death. "The bottom line is, this ain't all there is," he says. "If it *was* all there is, it's probably a realistic expectation to see it as catastrophic. But it's not like I'll never see Karen again; it's not like there isn't life after death."

That kind of understanding, even in the midst of our grief, can make a huge difference in how we view death. However, the reassurance of someday being reunited with that person in heaven is not the only comfort that God offers us.

Janaha experienced comfort from God in a variety of ways. As she spent time privately praying, reading her Bible and journaling while her mother was dying, she received comfort through the Scriptures, especially through the many psalms in which David cried out to God and God answered him. During those times, alone in her room, she also experienced God's voice speaking to her.

> I was hearing him say endearing things, reminding me that I was his daughter and that he was going to take care of me and that I could rest in him. I felt him pulling me close to his chest and telling me, "It's going to be OK, Janaha." I heard him continually say, "You've got to keep going; you can't give up." It was a lot of comfort, a lot of tender compassion. And I learned that he *had* a voice and that I *could* hear it and that I *could* be changed by it.

Janaha received comfort from God after her mother died, as well as before. While caring for her mother, she hadn't allowed herself to feel tired. She had often prepared her mother's meals, moved her (with help from her father) from the bed to the wheelchair and back to the bed, and even bathed her. But after many long months of waiting on her mother, she prayed, "I'm tired, God. I can't do this any more." God soon lifted that burden from Janaha and released her mother from her suffering. As Janaha grieved, images of her dying mother lingered in her mind. But God comforted Janaha in ways that counteracted the images—for example, by enabling her to see her mother as a role model of faith and servanthood.

We, like Janaha and John, can experience God's comfort in the midst of our grief over the death of a loved one. We can find comfort in knowing that Jesus is the resurrection and the life and that for those who know him, death is only a transition that separates us for a while. But we can also find comfort from him moment by moment as he answers our prayers and expresses his love to us.

### Struggling with Our Fears About Dying

Karen was a gift to me from God. It was 1974, and she became my first friend after I'd moved alone to a new city. I grew to love her for her thoughtfulness, her spontaneity, her sense of humor, her deep faith, her vulnerability, her sensitivity and her compassion. God used her to give me a sense of belonging at the church that we both attended and in the community.

A year after meeting Karen, I moved a few cities north to be near my future husband. And as often happens to friends, Karen and I let our friendship slide. Fortunately, she also fell in love, and she and I participated in each other's wedding. But we rarely saw each other after that.

When Karen called at Christmastime in 1980 to tell me she had been diagnosed with breast cancer in October and had had a mastectomy, I felt I had let her down. She was my friend. Why hadn't I stayed in touch with her so that I could have been by her side at a time that she most needed her friends, just as she had been at my side when I needed friends? I tucked my feelings into a dark, neglected corner of my heart and told myself to do better.

But the situation got worse. Both situations, actually—Karen's attempts to be rid of the cancer and my lack of response toward her. Although I again neglected to stay in touch with her, she called me the following spring with shocking news: recent tests had revealed that the cancer had returned and had spread to her lungs.

This time I didn't bother making promises to myself. Instead, I snatched the calendar off the wall and invited Karen to bring her family over for dinner. When they came, I took a few photos of Karen and her husband and their two-year-old daughter, and although I often took photos of friends, I knew that I was doing it because it might be my last chance.

But I called Karen only once after that evening. "Well, *when I feel better,* we'll get together," she said in a "let's pretend" tone of voice. However, I was emotionally paralyzed throughout the following summer and then into the fall, in spite of my almost-daily attempts at self-talk. I usually tried a positive approach: *Don't worry about past failures; just call her today and ask her how she's doing.* When I finally realized that trying to erase the past wasn't working, I tried a scare tactic: *One of these days you're going to get the phone call you've long dreaded, and it will be too late.* But still I did nothing.

One chilly day in November 1981 the dreaded phone call came. It was from a mutual friend, Sherry. Karen had died the day before. She was thirty-three years old.

I grieved deeply over losing Karen, and my heart ached for her daughter, who would probably grow up with no conscious memories of her mother. I also grieved over lost opportunities to tell Karen how much I loved her and valued her friendship. I felt guilty about that. And yet, despite my guilt, God didn't allow me to flog myself. He kindly set the guilt issue aside for a later time, when I would be ready to face it and to receive his healing.

As the time arrived, God showed me that what had paralyzed me was my inability to deal with loved ones who are dying. All my life I had been sheltered from death, and I was fortunate that no one very close to me had died. Until Karen. Following her death, God led me to a dark corner of my heart to discover what was hiding there.

First, I recognized my persistent denial. An irrational part of me was holding on to the childish belief that no one I loved would ever die. I gave that realization to God and repented of lying to myself.

Next, I identified several fears—the fear that death is real and permanent and unfair, the fear that it could happen to someone I loved, the fear that the dying process would be hard to look at and accept, and the fear that breast cancer or some other insidious disease could happen to me just as easily as it had happened to Karen. Although the fears were not wrong in themselves, I had allowed them to control my life. I gave those to God as well and repented of not trusting him for the future. Knowing that God had forgiven me, I was then able to forgive myself.

In 1996 I crossed the final frontier of my unresolved feelings about Karen: an underlying feeling of regret about my inaction toward her. I still longed to turn back the clock to 1981 so that I could call Karen frequently, visit her, read to her, fluff her pillows, make her something to eat, run errands for her and pray daily for her. (Yes, I had sometimes neglected to even pray for her.) I also yearned to tell her how her friendship had saved me from months of certain loneliness and had changed my life forever.

My inaction, rooted in a fear of the unknown, was understandable. Yet I knew that the regret could paralyze me in friendships with others who might die of cancer. My biggest fear was that I would abandon another friend who was dying, just as I had abandoned Karen.

As I prayed and journaled about the regret, God talked to me about the separations, or divisions, that are caused by death. We who are Christians have heaven to look forward to after death, but that fact does not keep us from grieving over the physical separation caused by death. Likewise, the process of dying sometimes results in emotional divisions between the living and the dying. While death was a physically and emotionally agonizing process for Karen, it was also painful for me because of my fears. So painful, in fact, that I unconsciously allowed it to divide us.

In the time that followed, God led me through a process of prayer, journaling and Scripture reading that closed the gap that I felt with Karen, freed me from my fears associated with dying and gave me confidence that I could remain a loyal friend to someone who was dying. God's light had illuminated that dark corner of my heart. Healed, comforted and no longer bound by fear, I soon became close friends with others who had cancer, and I remained close to some who later died.

Many of us have similar regrets, and perhaps guilt feelings, about loved ones who have died, and we wish we could go back in time and show them how much we truly loved them. While we can do nothing to change the past, we can have our hearts freed from our regrets, guilt feelings and fears about death and dying. Just as God invites us to come to him with all of our other feelings, he also invites us to come to him with our feelings about death. Whether our actions—or, as in my case, inaction—involved some true guilt, God wants us to tell him about it. "Come to me, all you who are weary and burdened," Jesus said, "and I will give you rest" (Mt 11:28).

We can unburden our souls by praying privately, but sometimes our souls get the message more clearly when we do something outward. One effective means is to write out our prayers in a journal or note-book. Journaling can help us to articulate and sort out our feelings, present them to God and prepare our hearts to receive his responses. Another means is to acknowledge our feelings (including any guilt feelings) to a trusted church leader or Christian friend and ask that person to pray for us in our presence and to proclaim God's freedom and forgiveness to us.

The psalmist says that God "heals the brokenhearted and binds up their wounds" (Ps 147:3). Jesus is our Redeemer—the one who redeems our regrets over lost opportunities, takes away our fears and fills our hearts with forgiveness and comfort and hope.

### Receiving New Perspectives from God About Death

Having our fear of death replaced by comfort and peace from God is only the beginning of how God can change our feelings about death. The Bible promises new perspectives on death—perspectives that are full of hope and joy—for those of us who believe that Jesus died for us and rose from the dead so that, by faith, we can live with him forever. But because our old perspectives on death are deeply engrained within us, receiving new perspectives, like receiving comfort and peace in place of fear, may take time.

Joan has struggled for several years with whether she will die of breast cancer. She doesn't understand why God has allowed her to endure recurrences and various treatments for so long, and yet she wants to be content with not understanding his reasons. She has often prayed, "Lord, I'm doing everything I can do, and the rest is up to you. And maybe what you've got in mind for me is not what I want, but I need to accept your ways." Some days she finds it easier to pray that prayer than other days, because she deeply desires more time on earth. And so she also tells God, "I know that you're all powerful and that you could stop this from happening. And I still believe that you can do a miracle in my life."

Because she was young—thirty-eight at her first diagnosis—and all three of her children were still at home, Joan felt anxious for a while about God possibly allowing her to die, especially when she was also the primary caregiver of her mother. Eventually she gave the matter to God. "OK, Lord, if I'm not here any more," she said, "I know that somebody else in my family needs to take care of her, and I don't know who, but I'm going to trust you to work that out. I can't carry that burden any more."

God has responded in some other personal ways to change Joan's perspective about death. One of those ways was by a vision, or mental picture, that he gave her one day when she and some family members gathered for prayer before she was to be hospitalized.

> I was kneeling on the floor, and they had their hands on me while we were praying. And when we were through praying, I all of a sudden had a very powerful vision, almost like Christ praying with his disciples. And I had a feeling of oneness with Christ—that he understood what I was going through. He was asking for the cup to be removed, and he pleaded with God.

Joan still pleads with God to remove "this cup," she says. And she still finds it very hard to say, as Christ did, "Your will be done." But she prays that prayer every day, asking God to do his will in her life and to keep her from fearing what his will might include. God's gift to her of being able to identify with Christ in facing death has strengthened her to accept the uncertainty about her death.

Janaha found that her new perspective on death developed both before and after her mother died. God had already done enough healing in Janaha's heart that she was able to confidently stand up in front of a large group at her mother's memorial service and speak. God further healed Janaha when she found out that her mother had died with a smile on her face and her arms over her head, "as if she had reached toward something"—which until then her mother had been too weak to do in the last few weeks of her life.

After her mother died, Janaha also sensed God's reassurance that her mother was all right and that some good would result from her mother's death. "So finally, there was rejoicing," Janaha says. That comfort and eventual joy greatly changed Janaha's view of death.

> Watching my mother cross over has made death more evident in my life, of course, but it's also made death more beautiful, in a way. There is that peace that's still alive within the word *death*, because it's not final. Death was a life-giving thing for me through the grieving process after I lost my mother.

Janaha's grief, which included a bout of depression, has lessened as she has continued to receive God's comfort and more of his perspective. That perspective includes seeing the good that God has brought about through her mother's death.

I was praying back then for God's will to be done and for my mother to be in Paradise and that he would direct me in wherever I was supposed to go from there. And I think I've been seeing God answering those prayers even to this day. My life has changed so much since then, and I see how much my mother's death has empowered me to pursue the things that I need to pursue.

I still pray for help, and God continues to help me, provide for me, show me and love me. He's brought a lot of healing from the depression that resulted from the pain and grief over losing my mother.

Janaha's life has dramatically changed as a result of her mother's death, and Janaha's ways of looking at death have dramatically changed.

Margaret also has received new perspectives from God about death—especially her own. When she found out that she could expect to die from her recurrence of breast cancer, she and her husband met with their pastor. Margaret was deeply touched by his response to her.

He said, "As the shepherd of this flock, I realize the necessity of our people learning how to die well. We need to know how to die well, as Christians, because it's a part of our witness." And I thought, *What a revolutionary concept—that I might actually be able to teach others how to die!* So my response was, "Lord, help me to know how to die well. Please show me what that means." And I think he's doing it. I'm catching glimpses of it.

To "die well" means, for Margaret, to be faithful to God even with her final breath.

It's one thing to be faithful when I'm on my feet and feeling well, but I want to be faithful when I'm really sick. That will be the real test; that will be when I'm the weakest. And if I've prepared my spirit to submit to the Lord in that weakness, then I'm relying on him to do his work to preserve my witness. When I'm in a place physically where I may not be able to control all that I am—I may not be able to pray any more, for example—I believe God will cover that for me.

Margaret looks forward to being in the presence of God. She has been studying what the Bible says about heaven, and she's gaining a new perspective that helps her to cope with the fact that she's dying. Margaret says she has "a newfound understanding that I'm a spiritual being that happens to have a body, so that when this body is gone, it's no longer serving its purpose for me. I will still go on in a new and better way. When you look at it from that perspective, there's no need for fear."

This new perspective does not mean, however, that Margaret has no qualms about the effects of her death on her family and friends. She grieves over leaving them and identifies with the apostle Paul when he says he's torn between wanting to be with Christ and wanting to continue serving the people he loves (Phil 1:22-23). But like Paul, Margaret sees her hope as an anticipation of being in the presence of God.

> I have the hope of heaven. It's real; it's becoming tangible to me. And I talk about it very seldom, because it's selfish. While all the people who love me are grieving, it's insensitive of me to be too happy about the fact that I'm going to be in a much better place, because they *won't* be. Although they will be celebrating the release of this spirit from this body for me, it will be difficult. My hope of heaven isn't an escapist thing. It's not a hope just to get me out of this diseased body. It's not that I'm going to get rewards or that my body is going to be new. I'm beginning to see that the real power of it is that I'm going to be in the presence of God. And that I'm going to know him.

We can receive new perspectives from God about death and dying when we begin to see ourselves as spiritual beings whose bodies are only temporary. "When the perishable has been clothed with the imperishable, and the mortal with immortality," Paul says, "then the saying that is written will come true: 'Death has been swallowed up in victory'" (1 Cor 15:54). This means that God will someday give us whole, healthy bodies that will last for eternity.

Knowing and believing these things, however, does not automatically vanquish our fear of death. If it did, we probably would feel less dependent on God—and as Margaret says, knowing God and being in his presence is our greatest hope. We need to come to God with our fear, believing that Jesus, through his own death, conquered death, the ultimate enemy. "He will swallow up death forever," Isaiah said of the Messiah, hundreds of years before Christ was born. "The Sovereign LORD will wipe away the tears from all faces" (Is 25:8).

The fact that God looks at death in a much more hopeful way than we usually do does not mean that death is a trivial matter to him. If that were true, he would not have allowed his Son to agonize in the garden and then to suffer a criminal's horrific death on a cross. Nor would Jesus have wept over Lazarus's death, while knowing that he was about to give back to Lazarus a few more years of life. "Precious in the sight of the LORD is the death of his saints," said the psalmist (Ps 116:15). Jesus weeps. God the Father weeps. But they weep out of compassion—they weep because we weep—and not because death is something to fear, something that will separate us from God. "For I am convinced," said Paul, "that neither death nor life, neither angels nor demons, neither the present nor the future, nor any powers, neither height nor depth, nor anything else in all creation, will be able to separate us from the love of God that is in Christ Jesus our Lord" (Rom 8:38-39).

Although we all know we must die sometime, we'd rather it not be from cancer, and we'd rather it not be soon. But God does not want us to live in the fear of death. He wants us to cry out to him in our fear and dread of death. When we trust him, express to him our honest feelings and watch for his responses, the God who has defeated death will set us free from our deepest fears.

# 14

## SEEING OUR RELATIONSHIPS IN NEW WAYS

Whearen we're diagnosed with a life-threatening disease, our relationships take on new meaning. And as long as we survive, even if we're not currently fighting cancer, that new meaning doesn't go away. We see our husbands, our families, our friends—perhaps even our grumpy mail carrier or our neighbors who play country-western music at full blast—differently. We see them with new eyes. God's eyes. And we can be grateful for the ways that God has changed our ability to see them.

### Seeing Our Husbands in New Ways
We all know of marriages that fell apart not long after a crisis hit. In many cases, the marriage was already as unstable as a sand castle, and the crisis was the windstorm that blew it away. But even if our marriages are made of concrete, a diagnosis of breast cancer can be a jackhammer that breaks up the marriage into useless fragments.

However, the opposite can happen—and often does. As discussed in chapter nine, the strain that breast cancer often puts on a married couple can ultimately strengthen their marriage. Margaret, for example, found that her husband, Chuck, grew spiritually after Margaret's recurrence and also began to take more responsibility. Because the cancer had spread to Margaret's spine and hip joints, she had trouble walking, so Chuck installed a railing for their staircase. He also bought a cellular phone that he could take with him everywhere, in case Margaret needed to reach him on a moment's notice. Although Margaret is glad to feel so well protected and well provided for, she's just as pleased to see such maturity in her husband.

> I see these things as just the beginning of the process that God is working in his life. And he's building a stronger man—a man who is going to be better equipped for whatever the Lord has in store for him. So I see that what's happening to me is impacting my husband in a positive way that would not have happened any other way. And I love it!

Of course, for God to work so dramatically in Chuck's life, Chuck had to first make some conscious choices. In addition to the agreement that he and Margaret had made to forgive each other for past offenses, Chuck had adopted a different attitude from the one he'd had eight years earlier, after Margaret's first diagnosis of breast cancer. At that time, he didn't take her cancer seriously, he says, because he felt that medical treatments would cure her. "I didn't support her as much as I should have," he says, "because I was busy with my own life and I just didn't realize the way and the amount that the cancer affected her. And that's to my own shame."

Chuck was devastated by the news that Margaret's cancer was back and that she wasn't expected to survive. But that news led him to a life-changing decision.

> I promised her—and myself—that I would not abandon her like I did the first time. So every doctor's appointment, every treatment, I was there with her so that she wouldn't feel alone.
>
> Cancer is a disgusting disease. It's not at all predictable, it robs people of their dignity, and it destroys hope. It's the opposite of everything that God stands for. My desire in this experience was to humble myself and allow God to act. Only God can bring good out of bad. I want God to use this for his glory however he sees fit.

Like Chuck, Perry has supported his wife, Viola, in ways that he wasn't able to support his first wife when she had breast cancer. And he's grateful that God has given him a second chance. Viola was given no hope of survival unless she could qualify for a stem-cell transplant. But Perry's desire to marry her added to her reasons to fight for her life. "He said he didn't care if we had twenty days or twenty years; he wants whatever time we have together," says Viola. "We've passed the twenty days, so that leaves only the twenty years, and with God's help I'm going to give it my best shot."

Divorced when her four children were young, Viola credits Perry for teaching her that "marriage is a good thing." God has been the center of their relationship from the beginning, she says, and dealing with the cancer and the treatment has brought them closer together. They have discovered that "we are very good for each other in crises as well as when things are going along smoothly." Viola describes her feelings about Perry:

> Since I was already fighting recurrences of the breast cancer when I met Perry, I'm sure I see him differently from how I would have if I had not had cancer. I realize that he is a very special person, given to me by God. I have now experienced what a good Christian marriage is. I so appreciate everything he does for me, which has been an awful lot, since my energy level has kept me from doing all I need to do here around the house. I feel so honored that he loves me so very much and that he loves me, the person, and never notices the "missing parts." The love I have for him is beyond description; I have never loved the way I love him. There is a fulfillment in my life now that I have never known. I am so thankful for him and to God for putting us in the right place at the right time. I'm thankful that we were such good friends and that we enjoyed each other's company before we realized we loved each other very much. We really like spending time together.

As difficult as our cancer experience can be for our husbands, they also can experience some lifelong benefits. Karen, assuming that her husband would remarry, gave John a list before she died of things to "fix" about himself "for next time."

> One of the things she said was, "Lose the show-must-go-on attitude." And that was very true about me, because I was still teaching adult Sunday school even though my wife was very sick. But I'd made those commitments, so I did them; you know—"the show must go on."

Since her death, I've made fewer commitments. I've narrowed the things I'm willing to do in the context of the church community, the things I'm willing to do as an employee, the amount of time that I'm willing to put up with what I judge to be stupidity in business relationships. I tend to be a lot more real; when I feel something's important to say, I say it. I've taken the "lose the show-must-go-on attitude" thing to the point where I now say, "What show?" and "Go on?" If it falls apart tomorrow, I'll do something else. Life is too short to put up with that. The show *doesn't* have to go on.

Now, nearly twenty years later, John and his second wife, Nan, are benefiting from the changes John has made. Once, when John had begun a new job in a city two hours away and he and Nan were about to move their family there the next weekend, John realized that the job wasn't working out as he had hoped. They immediately canceled their plans to move, and John served notice to his new employer. He has never regretted that decision. And he attributes his ability to make that decision to his experience with Karen's cancer.

Many married couples feel closer to each other as a result of their experiences with breast cancer. Jane's comment is typical of the women I interviewed. Married for seventeen years when she was diagnosed, she and her husband found that her cancer "helped us to treasure each other more."

After I had breast cancer, I was often asked by friends if the experience had strengthened my marriage. "Not really," I answered, unable to imagine how John and I could possibly have been drawn any closer to each other than we were before my diagnosis. As I gained more perspective, however, I realized that our marriage had been strengthened in some subtle ways. While it hadn't changed how John and I related to each other, I was more confident about his complete acceptance of me no matter how I look or feel. In addition, I felt more confident that our marriage will survive any future crises—and I know they will occur. Despite the terror that I felt when I was diagnosed, I am grateful to God for my experience with cancer because of the greater confidence that he's given me through it.

Even the best marriages can be strengthened through an experience with breast cancer, as long as God is invited to be involved. We can be assured that, in contrast to the evil of the disease, God will give us good gifts through it. And if we're married, one of those gifts may be a greater closeness to our husbands.

## Seeing Our Children in New Ways

Although we naturally want to shield our children from our own fears and other negative experiences associated with our breast cancer, we know we can't. But God, in his generous love to us, often responds to those motherly fears by drawing our children closer to us and by giving them good gifts through their experiences of our breast cancer. Simple things mean more to them, for example. "It means a lot when I show up at the track meet—more than ever before," says Joan, whose ongoing battle with cancer has been a battle for her three teenage children as well.

Jane and her family were on a shopping trip while vacationing in Seattle, about a year and a half after Jane had finished her chemotherapy, when a necklace in a department store display case caught her eye. Made of sterling silver, the pendant had been cut in a circular pattern to depict a woman holding a child, and a card accompanying the necklace said, "A mother's love is eternal." As Jane read the card, she thought of her eleven-year-old daughter, Jenny. *I'll buy this, and I'll wear this all the time,* Jane thought, *and if I should die, Jenny will connect this necklace with me and with the message.*

So Jane bought the necklace and later showed it to her daughter. "Jenny, isn't this such a pretty necklace? The card says, 'A mother's love is eternal.'" Jane didn't say anything to Jenny about "if I should die," but Jenny, an affirming person normally, reacted with indifference.

Jane was puzzled. "Jenny, don't you like this?" she persisted.

Her daughter's response still reduces Jane to tears. "Mom," Jenny said, "I'd rather have *you.*"

Through that dialogue, Jane began to realize that her breast cancer ordeal, even though she herself no longer worried about it, had greatly impacted her daughter. Still present in her daughter's mind was the fear of losing her mother. And yet Jane's awareness of her daughter's fears, and those of her son as well, have benefited all of them by drawing them closer.

Janaha often had difficulty relating to her mother while her mother was dying. But she now realizes that God has used her mother's death to change how she values her other relationships.

> I've realized since my mother's death that there were a lot of things that were left unsaid and a lot of things that *I* could have said and ways that I could have cherished her. And that's made me want to be more of a compassionate, tender person to the people who are in my life now—valuing them in their lives and in whatever struggles they're going through. I don't value success too much. I don't value a lot of material things any more. I learned from my mom and my dad that there are more important things to worry about. I don't need a big, fancy car; my car is a blessing from God, and I pray every morning that it starts. I don't need to have a big, huge house, and I don't need fancy clothes and eighty-dollar shoes any more, and I used to like these things; I used to want them. But now I realize that people are more important. They're not going to wither away so quickly. It just makes more sense—family and community and relationship with God.

Janaha found that her perspectives about life and about God were radically changed by her mother's cancer experience in ways that became God's gifts to her.

> If my mother had remained alive and she didn't have cancer, I would probably not be who I am today. I probably wouldn't have come to a place with God so quickly. I most likely wouldn't have gone to Oregon to go to Bible college, where I had a great experience. My father and I wouldn't be having the relationship that we have right now. I wouldn't be living in the Santa Cruz Mountains. I wouldn't have the perspective that I have now. There's so much in my life that resulted from having gone through that experience—from the people I've met to the courage that I've had for doing other things in my life—and I'm thankful for it. When I get married, when I have my own children, all these different obstacles—or new experiences that *could* have been obstacles—will not be obstacles, because of my new perspective.

One of the Scriptures that Janaha held on to when her mother had cancer was 1 Peter 5:10-11: "The God of all grace, who called you to his eternal glory in Christ, after you have suffered a little while, will himself restore you and make you strong, firm and steadfast. To him be the power for ever and ever. Amen." Janaha feels that God has begun restoring her. "I know that in his grace he will reveal things within me and restore me, and as he does that, things will be made more clear."

We don't always know how our children or our grandchildren are being impacted by our breast cancer experience in either the short term or the long term. But we can be confident that God wants to bring about good results in their lives through the experience.

### Seeing Others in New Ways

Having breast cancer helps us to see our siblings, our parents, our friends, our pastors and church leaders, our coworkers and acquaintances and our health care professionals in new ways, as well as our husbands and our children. Viola has grown "even closer" to her mother, stepfather, brother and sister since she was diagnosed. And that was difficult, she says, because they were already her closest friends.

Bonita also comes from a close family. They have a long-standing tradition of gathering at her parents' house each week for Sunday dinner—Bonita and her husband and three daughters, Bonita's four brothers, her sister, and all their spouses and children, besides Bonita's parents. "In addition to that, we have lots of God-given brothers and sisters," says Bonita, "so it's no telling who shows up for dinner from Sunday to Sunday."

The entire extended family was shaken when Bonita was diagnosed with breast cancer in 1989. But when her mother was diagnosed four years later, Bonita felt that her brothers, in particular, were devastated. And yet she feels that God has brought good out of both her own and her mother's cancer experiences.

> "All things work together for good for those that love the Lord," and "what Satan means for evil, God means for good." That's the way that I look at things. So I feel like whatever the problem seems to be, some good is going to come of it. It's so strange to me that I had breast cancer at thirty-six and my mom had it at sixty-five. But did that make it easier for me to help take care of my mom? Yes. To know how to help her, to be there for her? Yes. To ask the doctors the right questions for her? Maybe. I'm sure my brothers were devastated with *me*, but they're so *close*

to my mother. They were praying! They knew that we already had that living testimony in our family, of what God had done.

Bonita's mother had always been the one to prepare Sunday dinner for who-knows-how-many guests. It was a lot of work, but she insisted. That is, until she was diagnosed with breast cancer. She finally gave in to her grown children, who began to take turns preparing Sunday dinner and have continued doing so. Bonita feels that the change in responsibilities has been good for her and her siblings, as well as for her mother.

It's not uncommon for a mother and daughter to share the experience of breast cancer firsthand. And it often draws them closer. Margaret's mother was diagnosed with breast cancer five years before Margaret, who describes how their relationship has benefited:

> When I went through breast cancer, my mom felt a new kinship with me and I with her. We had never been terribly close before, but since we have both been through breast cancer, we have been very close. And I'm very grateful for that. Now she's very actively involved in praying for me and expressing concern for me, because she's been there. She's a real support.

Margaret and her mother, who live several hundred miles apart, now have a "little five-minute check-in thing": her mother calls Margaret every morning at 7:15. "It's very helpful," says Margaret. "It makes us both feel in touch."

Most people don't have immediate family members who have had breast cancer. But if you asked them, most people would probably say they're personally acquainted with someone who has had breast cancer. And in most cases, their lives no doubt have been affected in some way as a result. This can be due to their own realization that life is fragile and that cancer can happen to anyone. But it can sometimes be due also to ways that those of us who have breast cancer see them differently. Whether they're close friends or they're casual acquaintances through work or church or the community, they may feel more valued because we have shared with them some aspect of our personal crisis. Viola and Perry were touched by the responsiveness of the people they met when they went looking for a new church. "The people there have been very supportive and have made us feel like we've been there for a long time," says Viola. "There is a genuine caring, and we feel we've found our church home."

Viola also realizes that her several recurrences of breast cancer and her experiences with doctors, which ranged from wonderful to horrendous, have enabled her to see her relationships with her current doctors in new ways:

> Because of the problem I had with one doctor, who said I was cancer free when tests performed later that day by my primary-care doctor confirmed that the tumors I saw and felt were malignant, it's been very clear to me that it's important for each of us to know as much about our illness and treatment as possible, so that we'll be aware when things are not right. I know the doctors I have now are good. I trust them because I've looked into their backgrounds and at their results with other patients. I feel very confident in their care, and I know they're concerned about me and my health.

Many of us have found that when others learn we've had breast cancer, they suddenly quit talking and start listening to us, often communicating a sense of awe about us. Joan is one example:

> I've had very good relationships built through acquaintances and a lot of my clients, and it's been very good. I've had many opportunities to share with people what God has done. And they tell me that I don't even have to say it—that they just know it by how I live my life and by my whole outlook. And that's been really good. I have a tremendous number of relationships with people in my community and everywhere.

Breast cancer is painful to everyone who is affected by it. But just as we can benefit from our experience in some ways, others can benefit from it too. As we begin to see each other more clearly, with God's eyes, we are drawn closer together, so that we all can be drawn closer to God.

# 15

# RENEWING OUR HOPE

Having breast cancer is often a roller-coaster ride of hopes—some that are raised and others that are so quickly dashed that our hearts leap into our throats. First, we hope that the doctor is right about the lump or the "atypical" mammogram and that it's "nothing to worry about." Then everything we've ever hoped for about our earthly lives dissolves as we hear the word *cancer.* Next, we hope that we're being cared for by the most expert doctors available, that whatever treatment we've chosen works and that neither the cancer nor the treatment will kill us. We also hope that we can soon function again on a normal level, preferably in a few weeks rather than months. And we hope that our families and friends will listen to us, love us and help us. Between all those hopes are some occasional disappointments: a treatment doesn't work as fast as expected, our oncologist pooh-poohs our report of a side effect, or a friend tells us the latest theory on why we got cancer. And underlying all these hopes and disappointments is the greater hope—perhaps the desperate, death-defying hope—that God hears our cries, understands our needs and plans to help us.

### Remembering Our Desperate Hope

Judy had suffered suicidal depression before her diagnosis. But her strength to hold on to God came partly from Hebrews 6:19, "We have this hope as an anchor for the soul," and Hebrews 10:23, "Let us hold unswervingly to the hope we profess, for he who promised is faithful." Her hope was grounded in God, so that she never felt that she was falling from the edge of a cliff.

Nancy, who has had a recurrence, sees her hope in the context of eternity:

> The statistics are so intimidating and the horror stories so prevalent. Being a believer allows me to stand on the hope of spending eternity with Jesus should the worst-case circumstance apply. Being a believer also allows me to cling to the hope that I may be totally and completely healed should the Lord desire that.

There is nothing wrong with hoping for God to completely heal us. Probably every woman I interviewed made that request of God many times. But those who haven't received a yes answer do not feel that either God has ignored their request or their hope is in vain. Instead, they talk about their hope in God—in his faithfulness, his goodness, his love—and in his promise that he will be with them throughout eternity. Facing breast cancer more than once, along with its threats to many of her hopes and dreams, prompted forty-two-year-old Joan to do some thinking about hope—especially desperate hope.

> My first time around [she was first diagnosed at age thirty-eight], I felt like I was going to fight this and I was going to get on with life again and that this wasn't going to interfere with my life any more. Maybe twenty or twenty-five years down the road I might get cancer again, and I might die at the age of sixty-five of some sort of cancer, but I didn't think it was going to do anything like that to me as a young person.
>
> But with my recurrence, it was like, *Oh, wait a minute here. I could die.* So then I began to feel desperate—*What am I going to do? I've got to keep*

*myself going.* I had to come to those terms, knowing that my hope is in God, no matter what happens, and come to understand life as a journey, a preparation for eternity. And that is our hope.

Many of us can say that our experience with breast cancer was worthwhile, because of the ways that God increased our hope in him. That in no way means that we see our cancer as a gift or as a friend. It is still an insidiously evil disease that we know didn't come from God. But for many of us, God has changed our experience into a gift of hope. Here's what Rachel says:

> As hard as that experience was, when you wrap the whole thing up in one big package, it was a far more positive experience than negative. Now, I grieved the fact that I had this major change in my life. But it was a gift. I remember in one Christmas letter I referred to it as "that really dark, black time in our lives," and yet my prayer was that I would never forget it, that I would always remember it and draw on it in future years. And that has been there for me. So God kept his promises over and over again.

The Bible is full of references to God as our hope. "Those who hope in me will not be disappointed," God tells Isaiah (Is 49:23), and one of the psalmists says, "The LORD delights in those who . . . put their hope in his unfailing love" (Ps 147:11). To hope in God does not mean to hope that he will give us what we ask him for. To hope in God means to believe his promises that he will always love us, always help us and always be with us. No matter how much we've been disappointed in the past, no matter how often we've lost our hope, God wants to renew our hope in him.

### Seeing God's Purposes in Our Cancer

While we're focused on trying to function within the limits of our fatigue, nausea, pain and emotional distress, it's all we can do to maintain some form of communication with God. And we may therefore find it hard to hear anything from him about his purposes. But later, when we've survived the treatments and we've watched God act on our behalf, we're better able to reflect on our experience and to understand whatever he wants to show us.

"The LORD confides in those who fear him," says David (Ps 25:14). God does not keep a secret from us when he can show us more of himself and his love by sharing that secret. He gives us some clues in the Bible about his purposes in allowing us to suffer, and I believe that our breast cancer is included in the suffering that he refers to. Three of those purposes are mentioned in a passage of Paul's second letter to the Corinthian church.

*Learning how to comfort others.* Paul writes, "The Father of compassion and the God of all comfort . . . comforts us in all our troubles, *so that we can comfort those in any trouble* with the comfort we ourselves have received from God. For just as the sufferings of Christ flow over into our lives, so also through Christ our comfort overflows" (2 Cor 1:3-5, emphasis added). One of God's purposes in allowing us to have breast cancer is to help us learn how to comfort others. When we have received comfort from God in our suffering, he empowers us to become agents of his comfort for those who are facing fear, disappointment and other feelings that we ourselves have faced.

Joan received a call from a woman named Kari, whom Joan had met through her children's school. Kari was depressed, because she had lost her job and was also having difficulties with one of her children. She wanted to make an appointment for Joan to cut her hair, because she didn't want to face her regular hairdresser. "I look horrible and I don't want to explain to him what I'm going through," she told Joan.

During that hair appointment Joan listened compassionately as Kari told her story. Joan understood Kari's feelings because she had experienced similar feelings in her own crisis. She was able to comfort Kari, and as she does with most of her clients, she told Kari about ways in which God had comforted her many times throughout her cancer experience.

Kari listened. She recognized Joan's comfort as something that originated not from Joan but from God. Soon Kari, her husband and two of their teenage children were attending church regularly with Joan and George. In fact, when Joan and George were baptized, Kari and her husband were among the twelve people who gave their lives to Christ during the service. A short time later, two of Kari's children also committed their lives to Christ and were baptized along with their parents. Although Joan sees her cancer as something that happened because we live in a fallen world, she feels that God has repeatedly turned her cancer experience into something good, including the changed lives of Kari and her family.

Introducing others to Christ through our breast cancer experience is only one of many possible outcomes as we learn to comfort others. As far as I know, no one met Christ as the result of my breast cancer experience, and that may be true for most Christian women who have had breast cancer. But we need not feel that God isn't using us. For me, the phrase "leading someone to Christ" has a broader meaning than explaining the gospel and watching someone give her life or his life to Christ. Every time we influence another person to be drawn in the direction of Christ, whether that person already has a relationship with him or not, we are leading someone to Christ. If you say something to me that encourages me and makes me thankful to God, you are leading me (once again) to Christ. If I listen to you with compassionate understanding, which we both know comes from God, I am leading you (perhaps once again) to Christ. We are fulfilling one of God's purposes in allowing us to have breast cancer, because we are comforting each other with the comfort that we ourselves have received from God.

*Learning more about relying on God.* Another of God's purposes in allowing hardships in our lives, according to Paul, is to help us rely more on God, especially when circumstances are beyond our control. Paul's letter to the Corinthian church continues: "We were under great pressure, far beyond our ability to endure, so that we despaired even of life. Indeed, in our hearts we felt the sentence of death. *But this happened that we might not rely on ourselves but on God, who raises the dead*" (2 Cor 1:8-9, emphasis added). Paul and his fellow missionaries thought they were facing a death sentence, just as we may have thought we were facing a death sentence. But just as God met them in their worst fear—their fear of death—he has met us in our worst fear.

Judy looks back and sees the difference made by one passage of Scripture (also from 2 Corinthians) throughout her entire cancer experience.

> We are hard pressed on every side, but not crushed; perplexed, but not in despair; persecuted, but not abandoned; struck down, but not de-

stroyed. . . . Therefore we do not lose heart. Though outwardly we are wasting away, yet inwardly we are being renewed day by day. For our light and momentary troubles are achieving for us an eternal glory that far outweighs them all. So we fix our eyes not on what is seen, but on what is unseen. For what is seen is temporary, but what is unseen is eternal. (2 Cor 4:8-9, 16-18)

"Light and momentary troubles"? Momentary, perhaps, relative to eternity. But "light"? Paul and his fellow missionaries were *suffering.* And yet while they sometimes felt discouraged, they did not ultimately despair. Although their bodies were "wasting away," their spirits—their real selves—were becoming stronger. God proved, in the midst of their suffering, to be reliable, by not allowing them to be crushed, despairing, abandoned or destroyed. And he renewed their hope.

Our breast cancer experience has been neither light nor momentary, relative to our other experiences of life. But we have not been destroyed by it. Even if our bodies are wasting away, our real selves are becoming stronger as we rely more on God. And day by day our hope is being renewed.

*Giving others the opportunity to thank God.* When I meet another Christian woman who has had breast cancer, I'm often amazed to hear about the many people who prayed for her. I'm further amazed to hear how those people rejoiced and thanked God with her, not necessarily for progress toward her physical healing (although that's something to thank God for, it doesn't always happen), but for the ways that they saw God intervening in her life and in the lives of her family. The good gifts that God gives us in the midst of breast cancer always spread to those who are praying for us.

The apostle Paul points to the thanks that others give to God as another purpose in our hardships:

> He has delivered us from such a deadly peril, and he will deliver us. On him we have set our hope that he will continue to deliver us, as you help us by your prayers. *Then many will give thanks* on our behalf for the gracious favor granted us in answer to the prayers of many. (2 Cor 1:10-11, emphasis added)

As the one who raised Christ from the dead, God delivers us from the fear of death, even if he does not deliver us from physical death. And those who have prayed for us can join us in thanking God. Our deliverance does them good while also bringing glory to God.

*   *   *

Sherin saw several possible purposes in her breast cancer, some for her own benefit and some for the benefit of others. She often saw herself as a branch that was being pruned to become more fruitful, as Jesus describes in John 15:2. "I began to realize that God allows us to go through trials to make us better and stronger and to build our faith in him," she says. "There was a purpose to the nightmare I was living."

Following my own diagnosis, a couple of acquaintances ventured that perhaps God had allowed me to get cancer because he was trying to get my attention. That hypothesis stung me. I knew—and I knew that God knew—that he already had my attention, and I was frustrated that those acquaintances were raising questions about me that had no basis in who I was. But just in case God was trying to help me recognize some blind spots in myself, I asked him if those people were right.

I immediately received his assurance that I was paying attention to him and that there were other reasons that he had allowed me to have cancer. I was relieved. Exactly what those other reasons were was not clear at the time, but in the weeks that followed, God comforted me with his presence, with Scriptures, with words and pictures, with the beauty of nature and with the words or the presence of dear friends. As I found comfort, God brought me opportunities every day to tell other people what he was doing in my life.

Although God does not cause our cancer, he can use it as a way for us to identify with other people who are suffering. We can benefit by drawing closer to God and by developing more compassion for other people. Those who are undergoing a crisis, whether they know God or not, can receive God's comfort when we're willing to let God use us. When we suffer, we also learn new ways of relying on God. And those who have prayed for us can share the pleasure of thanking God for all he is doing in our lives.

God seems to enjoy revealing his purposes to his daughters and sons. Knowing his purposes is one way of renewing our hope in God, and that hope can strengthen us and sustain us for the rest of our lives.

**Expressing Our Gratitude to God**

To experience God in the midst of breast cancer means that we eventually have many good gifts to thank him for. To begin with, God answered us when we cried out to him. He assured us of his presence, he comforted us, and he gave us hope. He saved us out of hopelessness. "I will give you thanks, for you answered me," says the psalmist. "You have become my salvation" (Ps 118:21). Paul tells the Ephesian church to "sing and make music in your heart to the Lord, always giving thanks to God the Father for everything, in the name of our Lord Jesus Christ" (Eph 5:19-20). Our lives can become an expression of thanksgiving to God for everything he did for us while we had breast cancer.

For some of us, an obvious gift is that God has restored us to good health. Margo has been grateful, ever since her recovery, for every day that God has given her. And as her daughter entered college, Margo has been specific in thanking God. "This year I've been aware of just how much she needs me," says Margo. "She's had a very hard year; it would have been a lot harder if I weren't around. So I thank God every time I've had a phone conversation with her, that I'm here for her. I am *so* grateful."

Although neither Margaret nor Joan has been restored to health, they are grateful to God for their times of feeling good. Margaret experienced excruciating pain at times as a result of her chemotherapy treatments. "And now every day that I feel good is an explosion of gratitude when I get out of bed," she says. "Having been to those depths, to have a day when I feel good is a cause for rejoicing and gratitude and thanksgiving."

Joan has felt good for many months, despite having cancer in her liver, bones, spine and remaining breast. She has been able to continue her hairstyling business full-time.

> For as much cancer as there is in my body, I'm doing extremely well. I *look* well. People look at me and say, "Who would even know that you were sick?" And God has certainly blessed me that way. Every day, I have to thank him, because I don't have a pain I can't live with. Even the doctors ask me, "You don't have pain?" "No." "You're putting in a normal day?" "Yeah." "Wow!" And I give God the credit.

In the summer of 1998 Joan joined the Knot a Breast dragon-boat team of women who have had breast cancer. She wasn't well enough to paddle, but she beat the drum to set the rhythm for her teammates.

Besides thanking God for giving us health or some temporary freedom from pain, there are many related gifts that we can thank him for. Connie thanks God that throughout her cancer experience she never felt alone. She also thanks him that many of her friends told her during that time how much she meant to them. Margo thanks God for surrounding her with people who cared about her. "I can remember talking with someone and feeling like that person represented God to me," she says. And Judy thanks God for drawing her close to her mother, through the shared experience of cancer treatments, shortly before her mother's death.

Viola thanks God for continually giving her opportunities to share with others what he has done for her. "Whether it's one-on-one in the doctor's office, with a support group or with a large audience, I am grateful to him for these experiences," she says. As a breast self-exam facilitator, Viola helps others learn to check their breasts for any questionable changes. In that role as well, she gives God the credit for her survival and her hope.

Whether or not God blesses us to outlive our breast cancer, we can never repay him for his many generous gifts to us. But there is one way that we can demonstrate our gratitude to him, in addition to saying thank you. As Margo says, "I would pray, offering God all that I am and have and ever will be." Jane sees her regular workouts at the Y as an act of prayer, in which she offers her body to God. And Gerry speaks for many of us as she describes some of her responses to God:

> I still am expressing the gratitude that I think saved me through that experience. I have more life that I can contemplate, and I keep asking, "What would you have me do?" To focus my life differently is, I think, the deepest expression of gratitude—a changed life. I want to be God's woman until my last breath—until I'm with him. And I keep asking, "How can I do that?"

Margo and Gerry and many other women have realized what Margaret realized as she drove home after hearing her doctor's diagnosis: that God wants us to present our bodies—whether sick or healthy, mutilated or intact—as living sacrifices to him (Rom 12:1). We may not

172 / *DESPERATE HOPE*

think that he can do much with us, but that's his decision. All that we are and all that we ever will be belongs to him.

### Celebrating What God Has Done for Us

One of the psalmists wrote that those who go out weeping, carrying seed to sow, will return with songs of joy, carrying sheaves with them (Ps 126:6). If you grew up in an evangelical church, as I did, you no doubt heard that verse quoted mainly in reference to missionaries. Certainly the verse can apply to them, but I think it can apply as well to our own longings for God to bring some good out of our breast cancer experience. We can trust him to hear the longings of our hearts. He may not give us what we ask for—relief from pain, long life, the chance to see our children or our grandchildren grow up—but he promises us joy if we seek him. Even in the midst of grief, we can celebrate his gifts of joy.

For Bonita, every birthday is a celebration of the life that God has given back to her.

> I don't think I will ever be self-conscious about my age. After having cancer, I was so thankful for every birthday. I'm very pleased, having had cancer at thirty-six, to say I'm forty-four. It's like there's nothing greater that I could say, because when I was thirty-six and had cancer, I didn't know how many birthdays I would have left.

Bonita especially appreciates what God has done when she remembers the enormous fear that she experienced after being diagnosed. "That is what I went from—fear of what this might mean in terms of dying, and then being thankful for every day that I had." That change has been a cause for celebration for Bonita and her family.

Similarly, Margo celebrates every time she's present at an important event, such as her daughter's graduation from high school. "That means I'm here," she says. "Periodically, I beg God to give me more years. And every year that goes by, I jump for joy."

Jane and her husband celebrated the end of Jane's chemotherapy treatments with a family vacation. They drove toward Monterey, on the California coast, and on the way spent a night at a popular hotel that provided special amenities such as bathrobes. "That was a real 'pampered' experience," says Jane. As another celebration, Jane's husband bought Jane a picture with the caption "Great is thy faithfulness!" which they hung on their wall.

Bonita also celebrated the end of her treatments with a vacation. She and her husband took a cruise to the Caribbean. But in addition, she sees other people's celebrations as opportunities for her to celebrate what God has done in her life. Her sister got married when Bonita was undergoing chemotherapy, and so Bonita celebrated not only her sister's marriage but also her own ability to remain standing as one of her sister's attendants during the ceremony. Bonita recently participated in her parents' fiftieth wedding celebration, an event for which she also celebrated being alive so that she could help them celebrate. "I celebrate *everything*," Bonita says. "Everything is so important to me."

Janaha, who shared the responsibility as a teenager of taking care of her mother, had felt burdened in many ways as her mother began to die. She remembers reading Scripture verses about rejoicing in suffering, and thinking, *Yeah, right! Rejoice in this pain, in this struggle?* But she realized later, when her own struggle became less intense, that she was rejoicing.

When Elena's son was about to turn four, Elena decided to celebrate his birthday and all the practical help she had received from the mothers of other children that attended her son's school. So she invited all twenty-eight of the mothers, as well as their children, to attend the party. Elena's husband was stunned that so many women had provided help.

Gerry and her husband, Howard, hosted a big party to celebrate their twenty-fifth wedding anniversary two and a half years after Gerry was treated for breast cancer. The event was motivated partly by Gerry's experience with cancer.

> I wanted to have a blast and invite the world and make it a big thing, because I don't know that we'll be here on our fiftieth anniversary. We celebrated it in fine style, and it's still reverberating in our lives. I'm so thankful that we let ourselves have that gift. That was a big way in which I celebrated to kind of balance the loss with much joy.

Gerry believes as strongly in small celebrations as in big ones. She celebrates her return to good health by giving time to herself—reading poetry or writing letters or visiting with a friend. "Sometimes they're really small things, because I don't have a lot of strength," she says. Now in her late sixties, Gerry has had back problems for more than twenty years and needs to take life at a slower pace than most people do. But she celebrates daily by looking for ordinary sources of joy.

> I found this paperback book once: *14,000 Things to Be Happy About.*[1] It was a list that this woman had made of things that made her happy. And I thought, *What a great idea!* So I started my own list. I said to my husband, "I love to see a full moon on a clear night in the summertime." I can love the sound of a bowl of scrambled eggs going into a hot skillet—things like that. I now take a lot more note of *little* joys in life, and it adds to my pleasure in a way that I had never expected. So I recommend that to anybody—not as a quick fix, but to focus on the things that we find beautiful or that make us happy or content.

Like Gerry, Joan is celebrating some of the little joys in life. Tragically, her metastatic cancer has now reached her brain, damaging her equilibrium and blurring her vision, so that she depends on a wheelchair for easier mobility. Yet she has found great pleasure in some humorous moments with her family. On a recent vacation with her husband and their three young-adult children, Joan had to leave her wheelchair outside a retail shop that she wanted to visit, because the entrance was accessible only on foot. So her daughter led her into the shop while the men in the family waited outside, along with some other men whose wives or girlfriends were shopping. When Joan and her daughter went back outside, there was Nate, Joan's eighteen-year-old son, "riding" the wheelchair and "poppin' wheelies" in the street. Eyeing his mother, Nate jumped up from the wheelchair, raised his arms and drew gasps from the small crowd he had attracted when he shouted, "I'm healed!"

Although we don't need to laugh to experience joy, laughter is one of joy's many expressions. One of my own favorite activities is dancing. Not *going out* dancing. And not necessarily doing choreographed movements. I relate to David, who said to God, "You turned my wailing into dancing; you removed my sackcloth and clothed me with joy" (Ps 30:11). With all due respect to my Baptist roots, I find that there is nothing like exuberantly, spontaneously leaping into the air, in time to a rhythmic beat, to express joy.

But whether we laugh, dance, sing, play music, participate in a wedding, throw a party, take a vacation or enjoy telling our stories to others, it is essential that we celebrate what God has done for us. When we celebrate his involvement in our lives, we renew our hope.

### Seeing God in New Ways

As we experience God, our perceptions of him change. Not that our perceptions were necessarily wrong. But we see more of him. We begin to see how big he is, how powerful, how gracious, how loving. And we stand in awe that the Creator of the universe pays attention to our individual needs. Seeing God in new ways renews our hope in him.

"It's as though he's gotten into my head and pushed outward," says Margaret. She explains:

> He is infinitely bigger to me now than I ever imagined before. There's a sense of wonder and awe at his majesty and at his infinite immenseness. It's that amazing paradox, that he is immense and fills the entire creation of heaven and earth—he's bigger than creation—and yet he loves me and cares for me individually. That sense is becoming more comfortably at rest in my mind. I've been real incomplete in my understanding of God, and one of my goals is to learn more about who God is, in these months that remain. And to begin to understand how immense he is and yet how completely and thoroughly he is involved in my life.

Janaha has a similar view of God after experiencing his presence during her mother's illness and death.

> Losing my mother caused me to be in a place where I needed to call on God. That was a first step for me. And as I continued to call on God, he continued to bless me with an eternal perspective and his love and his guidance. And now everything I look at and every person that I interact with—it's different. Even the sky looks like it's a different color than it was before.

One of the ways that God changes our perceptions of himself when we have breast cancer is by giving us a greater sense of his presence. That was Judy's experience:

> I was newly aware of God as my constant companion, personally involved in the details of my life. My communication with God is more open and

honest—sharing feelings of anger or fear with him. If I include the other circumstances occurring in my life around my breast cancer experience—depression and my mom's death—this was probably the darkest time of my life. But God was the light in my darkness. My trust in God's faithfulness deepened and grew. God, who brought me through so much during this time, is with me in my present and future, working out his perfect plan for my life.

Our communication with God is influenced by how we view him. Gerry has always had a strong image of God as Father, and that image holds a deeper meaning for her now as a result of her cancer.

I see him as a loving Father who wants to put his arm around me and cradle me. I feel very protected with that image. And my experience made me more trusting in the goodness of God. I *know* he's good. I think he demonstrated his integrity—biblical truths like his longing for us and his tenderness toward us and his willingness to respond to us, his strengths to uphold us, which are far beyond any human strengths.

Gerry's communication with God has taken on a more personal style. "I have a more acute sense of who he is—that I *know* who I'm talking to," she says. "He's not somebody far off; he's real and personal to me."

God often uses our communication with him to show us more about who he is. One spring day, six months after my mastectomy, I walked alone toward an attractive San Francisco neighborhood about a mile from my home. As I began to cross an intersection, I noticed the driver of a small sedan pulling up to the stop sign. Her jaw was tight, her eyes were fixed straight ahead, and she appeared to be mustering every ounce of her energy to resist whatever would get in her way. I was moved to tears without knowing why. And then God seemed to say to me, "People are a lot harder on themselves than I am on them. They don't know the freedom that comes from redemption and release. Have compassion on them."

Pondering God's words and the woman's face, I entered the tree-lined neighborhood, which was dominated by overgrown, neglected gardens. The rain had been sparse that winter, and yet I saw arrays of brilliantly colored flowers everywhere that seemed to have a message for me. Suddenly the word *grace* resonated in my soul with every patch of cosmos, hydrangea or Icelandic poppies I passed. Up and down the sidewalks and over fences and broken-down trellises, the ubiquitous blossoms spoke *Grace! Grace!*

My joy was soon tempered by a deep sadness. I thought about all the years that I'd heard *grace* defined as "unmerited favor." But I realized that it's much more than that. Such "favor" can be devoid of intimacy, affection and devotion. True grace is what the Bible describes as "*glorious* grace"—the "riches" of God's grace, which he has "lavished" on us (Eph 1:6-8, emphasis added). And yet even those of us who have a relationship with God see only a glimpse of his grace, his compassion. The abundance of brilliantly colored flowers was far beyond what our rainfall would ordinarily produce, and God said to me in the gentle voice of his Spirit, "This is nothing compared with the grace that I want to pour out on my people—and on the people who will *become* my people."

I then remembered that prior to my diagnosis I had often asked God to give me more compassion. And I realized that he had used my breast cancer to answer that prayer, by demonstrating more of his compassion toward me. I remembered that when my childhood memories of nightmares under ether made me afraid of facing anesthesia for the surgical biopsy, God gave me a bouquet of fragrant herbs from a friend's garden as a promise that he would be with me. When I was afraid that a mastectomy would limit my range of motion in my left arm, he prompted an unwitting friend to read aloud in church,

> I have loved you with an everlasting love;
>   I have drawn you with loving-kindness.
> I will build you up again
>   and you will be rebuilt. . . .
> Again you will take up your tambourines
>   and go out to dance with the joyful. (Jer 31:3-4)

God assured me every day, by leading me to Scriptures or by speaking to my heart, that he was my strong refuge who loved me and would never abandon me. And he poured out his compassion on me through my attentive husband and through many, many friends. Along with receiving and learning compassion from God, I was also experiencing more of the God of compassion.

Shortly after my mastectomy, God led me to a familiar but mysterious passage:

> "No eye has seen,
>   no ear has heard,
> no mind has conceived
>   what God has prepared for those who love him"—
> but God has revealed it to us by his Spirit. (1 Cor 2:9-10)

God was broadening my understanding of who he is and all that he had done for me. And mysteriously, I began to realize that losing my breast was nothing compared with all that I had gained as a result.

When we were new to the experience of cancer, our joys and comforts were perhaps no more than consolation prizes. But after a while, as God revealed more of himself to us, those joys and comforts became something permanent, something priceless and enduring, that we will treasure for the rest of our days. We can point to each of them and say, "That was a gift from God." And we can point to God and say, "I know him better as a result of having breast cancer."

The prophet Isaiah says,

> Those who hope in the LORD
>   will renew their strength.
> They will soar on wings like eagles;
>   they will run and not grow weary,
>   they will walk and not be faint. (Is 40:31)

Our strength is renewed when we hope in God. No matter what breast cancer may do to our bodies, God strengthens our hearts so that we walk confidently, run passionately and soar at unimaginable heights. Fear has no hold on us. Our desperate cries are answered. Our darkness has turned to light. Our desires and our dreams rest safely in the heart of the one who loves us infinitely, the God of hope.

# *Epilogue*

## EXPERIENCING GOD TODAY

The women and men you have met in this book have far more to say about experiencing God as their desperate hope than could possibly be contained in these pages. Their stories have communicated hope to people they've met in their workplaces, their churches, their cities and their neighborhoods, as well as to their families and friends. Here are some updates on their lives. (You can assume that none of the women have had recurrences of cancer unless noted otherwise.)

*Bonita,* who was only thirty-six when she was diagnosed in 1989, continues to direct a program for the juvenile girls probation department in her county. She and her husband, Carl, and their daughters still have Sunday dinner each week with Bonita's extended family. Their oldest daughter, Erika, is in college; their middle daughter, Erin, is in high school; and their youngest daughter, Brittany, is in middle school. They live in Oakland, California.

*Connie,* at age fifty-four, was tipped off about her breast cancer in 1996 by a swollen arm that wouldn't return to its normal size. A resident of Santa Barbara, California, Connie and her husband have two grown children and four grandchildren. Connie enjoys working in her garden.

*Elena,* who chose to use a fictitious name, grew up in Monterey, Mexico, where she worked as a librarian and performed folkloric dance. Elena was diagnosed in 1996, at age forty-four. She lives in Belmont, California, with her husband and young son.

*Frieda,* who was forty-five when she was diagnosed in 1995, continues working as a medical technologist at a local hospital and singing in the choir at her church. She lives in Beaverton, Oregon, with her husband. They have two grown sons.

*Gerry* was sixty-four when she was diagnosed in 1993. She now serves as a volunteer with the chaplaincy program at a local hospital. After going off tamoxifen in 1998 and being released from any further oncology appointments, she celebrated by reading aloud Psalm 116—about God saving her from the threat of death—first to her children and later to her fellow chaplaincy volunteers, who responded to her with applause and hugs. Gerry and her husband live in the San Francisco Bay Area and have three children and four grandchildren.

*Janaha,* now twenty-three, recently became a bride. She and her husband, Luke, are living in Utah while they prepare to move to Greece, where Luke will attend seminary. Janaha has studied hand-weaving and enjoys working on her own floor loom.

*Jane* still enjoys her job as dean of students at Westmont College in Santa Barbara, California. Diagnosed in 1993 at age forty-two, Jane is grateful for the emotional support she received from the college community. She lives in Santa Barbara with her husband and their teenage son and daughter.

*Joan* died of breast cancer on November 3, 1998, after five and a half years of fighting to survive. A resident of Hamilton, Ontario, Canada, she was forty-three. Immediately following her death, her son Nate and two of his friends instituted an event at the Christian high school they attended—and where George, Nate's dad, teaches—to raise funds for breast cancer research. Inspired by Joan's vocation, they turned the high school gymnasium into a hair salon, and volunteers who had gathered sponsors had their heads shaved. They raised about ten thousand dollars.

Joan and George's daughter, Danielle, has her own apartment and is preparing for graduate school. Nate is now a university student, and their younger son, Josh, attends the Christian high school.

Joan had become my friend, and I miss her. But God has used her life and her death to convey to many people his love and compassion.

*John,* my late friend Karen's husband, age fifty-one, is a self-employed electronic engineer. Lori, the daughter born to John and Karen in 1979, is now a university student. John and his second wife, Nan, have another daughter, Rachel, who is in high school. They live in San Jose, California.

*Judy,* a forty-nine-year-old children's librarian from the Tacoma, Washington, area, feels that her breast cancer experience has prepared her for a closer relationship with her sister, who is being treated for stomach cancer. Judy has been writing a devotional book for people with chronic illnesses. She was diagnosed in 1994, at age forty-three.

*Margaret,* who was known to her friends as Margo, has received her deepest desire: to be with Jesus. After a surprising year-plus in remission, her metastatic cancer returned and spread quickly. In July 1998 she breathed her last breath in *Chuck's* arms, with her son, her parents and her two brothers gathered around her. She was fifty-two.

Chuck continues to live in the Portland, Oregon, area, where he works as an electrician. While he "misses Margaret terribly," he is being comforted by the many people in their church who love him and loved Margaret.

I will always be grateful that in my friend Margaret I saw more of Jesus and experienced more of his love.

*Margo* was diagnosed in 1989, at age forty-nine. She is a full-time therapist in private practice. She always looks forward to holidays, when her son and daughter come home from college, but meanwhile she enjoys spending time with her husband, stepchildren and grandchildren. Margo and her husband live in Saratoga, California.

*Nancy,* a technical secretary, was diagnosed in 1990, at age fifty-five. Although she had a recurrence nearly five years later, she now feels healthy. Nancy enjoys needlepoint, gardening, and singing in her church choir. She lives with her husband in Santa Barbara, California. They have a grown son and daughter.

*Rachel* enjoys working as a real estate agent and spending time with her children and grandchildren. Now sixty-three, she was diagnosed in

1981, at age forty-five. Although she had surgery for colon cancer in 1994, Rachel has had no evidence of cancer since then. She lives with her husband, Robert, in Ontario, California. They have three grown sons and eight grandchildren.

*Sarah* celebrated her forty-fifth birthday in early May 1999 and less than a month later, after becoming bedridden from her metastatic cancer, told her husband, Jonathan, that she was "ready to go home." God gave me the gift of saying goodbye to her in person a few hours before she indeed went home. Sarah and Jonathan's parents and siblings came from England to actively participate in a tearful but jubilant service of thanksgiving and worship.

Sarah and Jonathan had moved to San Francisco from London in 1993 with their two sons, Robert, now thirteen, and John, now ten. Sarah was diagnosed with breast cancer two years later. I feel privileged to have been one of Sarah's friends and to have experienced firsthand her reputation as a loving, giving servant of God.

*Sherin,* a single mother of two grown sons, continues working as an administrative secretary. She also volunteers as a trained *doula,* or labor companion, for mothers-to-be. Sherin was diagnosed in 1991, at age forty-three. She lives in Torrance, California.

*Viola* and *Perry* are delighted that God used the high-dose chemo/stem-cell transplant procedure in January 1997 to give Viola back her life. First diagnosed in 1982, at age forty-five, Viola had three recurrences and underwent several chemotherapy series before the stem-cell transplant. She still occasionally transforms herself into Iris the Clown and visits groups of children. She is also certified to teach breast self-exam. Viola and Perry live in Hemet, California, and have a blended family of seven children and thirteen grandchildren.

Each of us whose story is in this book has the pleasure of a full heart. As we continue to experience God—whether we're healthy or we still have breast cancer or we're in heaven seeing God face to face—we can say with David,

> Many, O LORD my God,
> > are the wonders you have done.
> The things you planned for us
> > no one can recount to you;

were I to speak and tell of them,
they would be too many to declare. (Ps 40:5)

Our hearts are full of gratitude to God for what he has done in our lives and for who he has been to us. Our hearts are full of love for him. Our hearts are full of hope.

# *Appendix A*

## FINDING
## SPIRITUAL
## SUPPORT

Talking with someone who has been there is crucial when we've been given our diagnosis and we want some help. There is no substitute for the reassurance, the encouragement, the hope that a person who has traveled the difficult road of breast cancer can give us, especially if she has experienced God's presence along the way.

If you have been diagnosed with breast cancer recently, you may find it helpful to join a cancer support group. If you simply want to meet other women who have cancer and their faith or their lack of faith isn't important to you, you should have no problem finding a cancer support group through a local hospital, medical center or cancer treatment center. Many medical organizations provide support groups as a community service, sometimes for free.

However, if you are looking to God for meaning and purpose in your illness, you will probably want to find a cancer support group that includes other women who are seeking answers from God. Two of the women I interviewed, Rachel and Joan, have led cancer support groups with a Christian orientation. That is, discussions of God and questions for him and about him were encouraged at their meetings, and time was always set aside for participants to pray for each other.

Christian support groups for women with breast cancer are not plentiful; it's easier to find a Christian support group for both men and women experiencing various types of cancer. Many Christian women who have had breast cancer have told me they wished that either their own churches or churches nearby had provided support groups for women with breast cancer or at least for women with cancer. Several women said they had tried support groups provided by local hospitals but quit going because the groups weren't helping them. "It was good to know that others had some of the same feelings, but they didn't quite meet my needs because I needed to know that God was still in control," says Sherin, who believes that the Christian community should provide support groups that meet needs with prayer.

Bonita, who did find a Christian support group for women with breast cancer, is disturbed that many churches focus on praying for healing for the sick and on providing practical help but do not deal with "the day-to-day question What does this mean?" Many Christian support groups, however, exist for the expressed purpose of seeking God for answers to such questions.

If your church doesn't sponsor a cancer support group, you might ask your pastor which Christian churches in your vicinity have *any* support groups. Then you can call those churches to find out if they have a group specifically for people who have cancer. If they don't, they may know where you could find the nearest one.

A word of caution if you've recently been diagnosed and you feel inspired to start your own support group: Don't do it. At least not now. Wait until you've completed all your treatments and you've had a few months afterward to gain an overall perspective and regain your energy. You need all your energy right now to get well.

You might be fortunate enough, however, to find two or more women who are willing to organize and lead a support group. I say "two or more" because one person should not take on the responsibility alone. Taking charge of a group of people who are suffering physically and emotionally—including some who may soon die—is a demanding and sometimes draining responsibility. In addition, coleaders need each other to share ideas and to help resolve issues that arise within the group. Both Rachel and Joan worked with partners and say that they would not have done it alone. A support-group leader needs at least a backup, if not an equal partner, to share the load.

## Establishing a Network

If your search doesn't turn up a cancer support group and you don't find anyone who wants to start one, I recommend the next-best thing: that you establish your own support network. Starting with your own church—providing, of course, that you still have a little energy—talk to several women church leaders and try to find out who within the church has had breast cancer. When you find them—and you may want to also ask among your friends who attend other churches—ask those women about their experiences. Ask them also what questions they asked God while they were fighting breast cancer and how God responded to them. Then ask if you may keep in touch with them by phone when you have questions or when you want to talk about your experience with someone who's been there. In this way you can create your own ad hoc, informal support group without anyone having to attend any meetings. And those women may become a lifeline for you.

Soon after her diagnosis, Jane, age forty-two, was at a restaurant when she recognized a woman in her seventies whom she had briefly met at a church sometime before. The woman reintroduced herself and told Jane that she also had had breast cancer at age forty-two, when recovery from breast cancer wasn't as common. "They thought I would die for sure," the woman told Jane, "but God has been good to me, and he's going to be good to you." Jane not only became more hopeful about her own condition but also began to discover that many women around her had had breast cancer.

After finding out about my own breast cancer in 1990, I called Margo, who had been diagnosed ten months before me. Margo was feeling much more hopeful by that time and was able to encourage me. Her breast cancer had been different from mine, but she had undergone a mastectomy, which I was reluctantly contemplating for myself, so she helped me to feel that I wasn't alone. In that conversation, Margo referred me to another woman, Katherine, who also had had a mastectomy, so I later received encouragement from Katherine as well.

Margo and Katherine were only the beginning of a lifeline that God had custom-designed for me, just as the woman in the restaurant was one of many women who encouraged Jane. Some of God's most gracious gifts to us are people who have already bushwhacked their way through the same dark jungle that now surrounds us.

### Receiving Help from Pastors and Church Leaders

Pastors and elders or other church leaders are in a position to be extremely helpful to us following our diagnosis. That does not mean that they need to personally meet all of the practical and spiritual needs that we express. However, if the church has a goal, as many Christian churches do, of taking care of its members, the pastor and church leaders normally assume responsibility for seeing that that goal is met. Therefore, a women's ministry, for example, may take charge of finding out what we need, but the pastor or other leaders will want to make sure that the women's ministry is in touch with us and that we don't fall through the organizational cracks.

If you recently have been diagnosed with breast cancer and you attend a church, your pastor will probably want to talk with you to find out how the church can help you. He or she may or may not suggest a meeting, so you may need to take the initiative to schedule an appointment. Then you can tell your pastor what you think you'll be needing that the church might be able to provide. Many women with breast cancer have requested special prayer gatherings that were organized by their churches. Other women have been visited in their homes by the pastor or other church leaders and were sometimes offered communion or prayer accompanied by an anointing of oil. Many women have also benefited from practical help, such as meals prepared and delivered or transportation arranged for treatments. These are things that are appropriate for you to request from your pastor, if you want them.

You may want to also talk with your pastor about your emotional and spiritual needs. How are you feeling about having breast cancer? What are your specific concerns? How has your diagnosis influenced your ability to hope for the future? How has your diagnosis affected your family so far? And how has your diagnosis impacted your perceptions of God and your relationship with him? A good pastor, wanting to know these things, will listen carefully to what you have to say and will rely on God's direction for how to respond to you. A good pastor will not immediately quote Scripture—especially not Romans 8:28, "All things work together for the good." Glib responses and quick-fix solutions, no matter how sincerely expressed, can make us feel that the other person doesn't want to know about our pain and is not interested in helping us carry our heavy load. And the fact that such a response comes from the mouth of a pastor does not mean that that response is from God. If your pastor doesn't seem like a safe enough person to discuss these questions with, you may want to consider looking for another church. But more likely, your pastor will want to hear whatever you want to say about how you're doing. A wise pastor will offer his or her help rather than quick, easy solutions.

Margaret and her husband, Chuck, were pleased with the support they received from the pastoral staff of their church. One associate pastor told Margaret that when he found out about her cancer, he "sat down and cried like a baby." He said, "I know that pastors are supposed to have all the answers, but I've discovered that usually people in your position have more answers than we do, and I'm anxious to see what you have to teach me."

Margaret appreciated his attitude of "coming alongside me and not positioning himself above me, but actually really empathizing with me and caring about me and admitting that he just wanted to be with me through this process, even though he didn't have any answers."

Margaret and Chuck's senior pastor met with them the same day that they had consulted with the oncologist. The senior pastor, who had the same attitude as his associate, encouraged Margaret and Chuck to be "real" with people in the church and allow them to be involved in their lives, even though the church was large and many of the people weren't acquainted with each other.

In addition to talking with you, your pastor and church leaders can also encourage the establishment of Christian support groups within your church. They need to be careful, however, not to suggest that you start one yourself. That would be like suggesting that a seriously injured person go start a hospital. As mentioned earlier, breast cancer support groups are more likely to be successful if they are organized and facilitated by two or more women who have already gone through the experience of breast cancer or who have worked with breast cancer patients and are in a relatively strong place emotionally and spiritually. If no one in the congregation meets those qualifications or is willing to start a support group, pastors and leaders can help you by trying to find out if any cancer support groups with a Christian orientation exist in your vicinity. If they do exist, pastors and leaders can lend their support by publicly endorsing the groups, helping to fund them and publicizing the meetings.

If no one in the congregation wants to organize a support group, pastors and leaders may be able to direct you to someone else in the church who has had breast cancer. For example, Bonita left her support group after two years because it was hard for her to be around people who were dying. So she let her pastor know that she is available to talk one-on-one with women who have breast cancer but who don't want to join a support group or who want to talk with Bonita as an additional resource. That arrangement has worked well for her, and she feels that a number of women have been helped that way. No doubt her pastor is glad that Bonita is available when women ask the church for help.

Although the organizational structures that we might look for when we've been diagnosed with breast cancer are not always convenient or accessible, we can find rich spiritual resources within our sisters and brothers in Christ. God has provided them as agents of his love and care for us, so that we don't have to face breast cancer alone.

# *Appendix B*

## FOR HUSBANDS: REAFFIRMING YOUR WIFE'S SEXUALITY

Our husbands can be our most important source of healing as we recover from any perceived loss of sexuality. If I've learned anything from my marriage to John, it's how deliciously satisfying it is to feel loved even when I feel unlovable. All of the married women I interviewed talked animatedly about the unconditional acceptance and love that they received from their husbands throughout their breast cancer experience. If you're a husband who's looking for ways to reaffirm your wife's sexuality during breast cancer, here are some hints from a few of the women:

> This is such a tender time. There's a need for tenderness on the part of the man toward the woman. Psychologically, with the physical changes in her body, he needs to affirm that she's still OK for him. Chuck has done that beautifully. He's always been right there with me emotionally, going through the process with me and affirming that physically I'm OK. He's not outside looking on, saying "Ooh, your body's different, and I don't think I like this." And there's no rush, no pressure. I really appreciate that. (Margaret)

You married a woman who has or had two breasts and many, many other qualities that made her special to you. Only a small part of that is changed now. She is still her same wonderful self, but she needs more tender, loving care right now. She needs to feel she still has worth, she still is attractive. Tell her. Laugh and cry with her. Discern when she needs the arm around the shoulder. Let her know she's loved for the woman she is, not for her breasts or lack thereof. (Nancy)

Be able to look at the area and scar without being repelled. Let her know she is the same person as before and is just as beautiful. Let her know that you love her and that the loss of a breast is not a big deal to you. (Viola)

Margaret's husband, Chuck, has learned through both of Margaret's experiences with breast cancer what a wife needs from her husband during such times:

Take as much time as necessary with her, to show her that you're going to be with her and not abandon her, and to support her and love her as much as possible. That's what I've vowed to do. The first time, I didn't think of it as a deadly disease, but now it's obvious that it is. And so, my marriage vows to her—"in sickness and in health, till death do us part"—are much more serious. I've always wanted to be a man of my word, and I've failed many times. In *this* area, I'm *not* going to fail. And it's made a big difference. You are a part of her, and I believe that in a spiritual and physical sense. It's important to God that you honor your partner, and that honors him.

Nancy had a bilateral mastectomy (both breasts removed) followed by reconstructive surgery. But she says she never felt diminished in any way because of no longer having her own breasts. She was also continually reassured by her husband that not having her own breasts made no difference to him. "I feel just as loved and cherished as I ever have," she says. "Perhaps more so when he kisses the place where the left breast used to be!"

If you're the husband of a woman who has breast cancer, you're probably already feeling helpless in many ways. So the idea of remembering a list of things to do to reaffirm your wife's sexuality may set your head spinning. But it's simple: Love her. Love her body as you love your own. Love her as a whole person. And tell her, in as much detail as you can, why you love her. That's all you need to do. And God will use you as a powerful gift of healing in her life.

---

**Here are a few suggestions for helping your wife regain her sense of sexuality after breast surgery or during other treatment:**

■ Invite her to talk with you about what she's experiencing. Ask her what she needs from you, and discuss what the two of you can do together that might help her.

■ Encourage her to talk with her doctor about any aspect of her sexuality that she thinks she has lost. If she's undergoing chemotherapy or taking other medication, her doctor may be able to identify the loss as a side effect and may have some suggestions.

■ Offer to pray with her about her fears or other feelings related to her sexuality and about any ways that your marriage is being affected.

■ If she's had breast surgery, be willing to touch the scar as soon as possible after the bandage is off, if she seems ready. During lovemaking, keep in mind that the scarred side needs love too.

■ Ask her specifically what still gives her sexual pleasure and what, if anything, to avoid. If you are afraid of hurting her—or if you have other fears—say so. Don't be afraid to ask her questions and to express your concerns.

■ Make a list of all the things you like about your wife's body and whatever else attracts you to her sexually.

■ Buy your wife a card that expresses your love for her, and leave it on her pillow.

■ If you like to write, consider writing an erotic poem or essay about your wife. Then surprise her with it when she's not distracted.

■ Discuss with your wife the possibility of setting aside a regular time to massage each other or to give each other a "love bath," with or without sexual intercourse. Physical caresses, both given and received, will play a vital part in helping her to feel more sexual.

■ Plan some romantic dates with your wife, away from home, whether it's a movie, a candlelight dinner, a stroll through your neighborhood on a moonlit night or a hike to the summit of her favorite mountain.

■ Do some spontaneous romantic activities away from home, such as driving to a romantic spot after dinner to watch the sun set or to gaze at the stars. While you're there, reminisce with your wife about how the two of you first fell in love with each other.

■ If you and your wife like to dance, put on a CD that you both like and invite her to dance with you. Include some long pieces that are good for slow dancing. Or plan a date for getting dressed up and going out dancing together.

■ Surprise her occasionally with a romantic gift—perfume, bubble bath oil, a bouquet of her favorite flowers, a sexy nightgown or a gift certificate for a facial, a manicure, a makeover, a new hairstyle or a massage. If you can afford it, plan a weekend getaway in a romantic place that includes a jacuzzi.

■ Remind her regularly of the many things you enjoy about her, so that she will be reassured that you see her as a whole person.

■ If you and your wife find it difficult to communicate about sexuality issues—even after you have tried some of the preceding suggestions—discuss seeking help from a counselor together. If your wife isn't willing to see a counselor, consider seeing one yourself.

# Appendix C

## HOW CAN I HELP A WOMAN WHO HAS CANCER?

As someone who cares about a woman who has been diagnosed with breast cancer, you probably share some of the shock, fear and other feelings that she's experiencing. You may feel frustrated that you are powerless to help her get better, and yet you want to do something for her. You immediately tell her that you were shocked to hear of her cancer. But what else can you do to express your care?

No matter what your relationship is to the woman—husband, daughter, other family member, friend, pastor or church leader, co-worker or acquaintance who wants to be her friend—there are many ways you can help her. This appendix discusses some suggestions and guidelines that have come from both the good and bad experiences of women who have had breast cancer.

**Listening Compassionately**
Listening compassionately when she wants to talk is one of the best ways you can help a woman who has been diagnosed with breast cancer. In any conversations you have with her about her cancer, consider first that she may want to talk about what she's experiencing. Face her

squarely and give her good eye contact—or ear contact, if you're on the phone. Let her know she has your full attention. Be gentle and brief in your responses to her. If you feel awkward and don't know what to say, tell her so. And ask her how you can best help her. She'll probably appreciate your honesty, and she may make some specific suggestions.

If she seems to be comfortable in discussing her cancer with you, she'll probably welcome some basic questions—for example, about what kinds of treatment she's considering. Ask questions based on what she has told you, perhaps using some of her words or phrases. For example, if she says, "I'm frightened," you might ask, "What is it specifically that frightens you the most?" Or ask questions based on your observations of her. For example, if she seems anxious as she tells you about an upcoming procedure, you might say, "You seem a little anxious. Are you?" Stay away from aspects of cancer that she hasn't already mentioned, however. She may not want to discuss such topics as possible side effects of treatment, alternative treatments, her projected life span and her family's future.

If she begins to cry and seems embarrassed by her tears, reassure her that you aren't bothered. (And if you *are* bothered, you might bear in mind that she will probably feel better if she cries.) If you are a man, resist the impulse to touch her while she cries, unless you know that she is comfortable with such gestures from you. Otherwise, you might gently put your hand on her forearm or on the back of her shoulder to communicate your care for her. If you are a woman but not a close friend, you might ask her if she would like you to hold her. But whatever physical expression you choose, be careful that she doesn't interpret it as an attempt to make her stop crying. People who are uncomfortable with someone else's tears sometimes try immediately to comfort the one who is crying. The self-consciousness of the one who is crying then turns to embarrassment about having made the other person uncomfortable, and that embarrassment turns off the tears. To prevent that from happening, you can tell her, as you reach toward her, to go ahead and cry and to take her time.

### Offering Practical Help

Women who have breast cancer appreciate not having to ask for help.

"You're already feeling vulnerable and helpless, and a lot of your dignity is being stripped away by doctors and procedures," says Margaret. "So if someone simply shows up and says, 'This is what I'll do for you,' it's a relief." Margaret's next-door neighbor announced to her that "from now on, when we mow our grass, we're mowing your grass." For Margaret that was a helpful gift, because she had bought a push mower to use for exercise and then had become too ill to use it.

Women who have breast cancer also appreciate specific offers of help. An open-ended offer, such as "If there's anything I can do . . . ," is usually unhelpful, because it puts pressure on the woman to determine precisely what the person means by "anything" and whether the offer is genuine. However, if you see a practical need in her life—transportation, errands, meal preparation, child care, gardening—and you want to help, tell her which specific need you would like to fill, and give her a choice of dates that you could do it. You might say, for example, "I'd like to bring dinner over sometime this week; which is better for you—Tuesday or Thursday?" or "Can I pick up a few things for you when I go to the supermarket this afternoon?" or "Tomorrow is my day off; can I drive you someplace?" or "Why don't you let me take your kids to the park on Saturday?" But be sure that your specific offer of help is appropriate to your relationship with her. If her children haven't spent much time around you, for example, she might turn down your offer to take them to the park.

If you belong to a church or other group that would like to help the woman who has breast cancer, consider organizing a team of people who could drive her to treatments or provide meals or housecleaning services for several weeks or months. But you needn't worry if you don't have time to plan your favorite menu. Gerry remembers with pleasure the friend who brought over a carton of hot soup from a local restaurant and a loaf of French bread. The friend apologized that the dinner was "so plain and simple," but Gerry told her later, "It was just what we needed. It was a wonderful gift."

It's important that you not assume that if the woman who has breast cancer looks and acts healthy, she doesn't need help. Judy, who lives alone and works as a children's librarian, was grateful that friends from her church didn't make such an assumption. She had just enough energy to continue working a full week while undergoing daily radiation treatments, but by the time she got home each day, she was too exhausted to prepare herself something to eat. Judy says she would not have been able to work if one of those friends hadn't arranged for meals to be brought to her every evening during the seven-week period.

### Offering Spiritual Help

If you are praying for the woman who has cancer, tell her so. She will probably appreciate hearing it, unless she is uncomfortable with expressions of faith. She will probably also appreciate knowing exactly what you're praying.

Prayers offered in person can be a significant source of encouragement to someone experiencing breast cancer. If the woman has other friends besides you who like to pray, you might offer to bring with you to her home two or three friends of her choice to pray for her. If you are a pastor or a church elder—or if both you and the woman who has cancer feel comfortable doing this without a pastor or elder present—you might also offer to share communion with her in her home. Be sensitive to the woman's need for rest, though. Bonita, for example, appreciated the women's prayer groups who occasionally called her and asked, "Could we come over and pray with you this evening? We won't stay long."

Women who have cancer usually appreciate reading Scripture verses that people send them, especially Scriptures that reminded them of God's love and faithfulness. Margo recently came across some pink cards on which her daughter-in-law had written Scripture verses and some lyrics to old hymns when Margo had cancer. "I used them every day," she says. And when Gerry told a cousin of hers, who had had breast cancer five years earlier, about her own breast cancer, her cousin said, "I'm going to have to send you back the Scripture that you sent *me*." To Gerry's amazement, a Scripture that she had sent her cousin was one that she herself had already turned to repeatedly during her own cancer experience. "So my gift to her," says Gerry, "became her gift to me."

If you are the woman's pastor, invite her to make an appointment with you and, if she's married, to bring her husband. When you meet with them, ask how the church can help meet their needs and the needs of their family. If they identify only practical needs, ask them about their emotional and spiritual needs as well. Although they may want to be reassured that God is in control of what's happening and that he cares for them, they won't need to hear a sermon. As a servant of God, you can probably serve them best by praying for them and by encouraging your congregation to be involved in their lives.

### Avoiding Unhelpful Ways of "Helping"

You'll want to keep in mind a few things to avoid as you try to help a woman who has breast cancer. But you can relax; most of the guidelines in this section are a means of merely relieving you of responsibilities that aren't yours.

*You are not responsible for cheering her up or making her feel good.* Any attempt to do so may make her feel that you don't understand the seriousness of her disease and that you're judging her for feeling bad about it—in other words, trivializing her experience. Ironically, one of the best ways you can help her to eventually feel better is to allow her to feel bad. If the people around her accept all of her feelings, she will more likely allow herself to experience the depths of her feelings now, which will help her later to receive God's gifts of peace and comfort.

*You are not responsible for assuring her that she'll be all right.* Some people try to convey hope by sharing their conviction that the woman is a survivor and that she will survive her cancer. But their words can sound hollow, because they have no more basis for believing those words than the woman herself has. Sarah was told by a few other people that she would be OK. "And it made me wince a bit," she says, "because I thought, *Well, I* might *not be.*" As it turns out, Sarah's cancer has spread to several areas of her body.

*You are not responsible for keeping the conversation going.* She doesn't want to hear about your aunt who had breast cancer, even if she's survived it for thirty years. However, if *you* have had breast cancer and the woman isn't aware of it, she'll appreciate hearing it, especially if you can convey hope to her.

Also, if you run out of things to say to the woman, don't avoid her.

She probably wants others to acknowledge that she has cancer and to briefly express their concern for her, but she also wants to be treated as normal. If she responds awkwardly when you mention her cancer and you suspect she doesn't want to discuss it with you, you might ask her if she would rather not be asked about it. If she does mind, she will probably appreciate your giving her the chance to say so.

*You are not responsible for determining what may have caused her cancer.* Despite the media's emphasis on reducing the risk of breast cancer, no study has ever proven that not doing the right things causes breast cancer. The last thing she needs is to feel that she's responsible for the battle raging in her body. And if she seems to have guilt feelings about it, you can reassure her that the cancer is not her fault.

*You are not responsible for curing her cancer.* Unsolicited advice, especially about the latest cancer "cures," is seldom appreciated. Sarah, for example, was deluged by offers of alternative remedies:

> Lots of friends said, "Try this, try this, try this." Ginseng. But I never tried it. And there was something to do with chilies as an alternative to chemotherapy. But I felt so right about taking chemotherapy. Somebody else gave me some kind of herbal tea. There was this stuff that looked like horse food, and I didn't try that either. And somebody else takes something that's like fruits and vegetables in a capsule. It's supposed to really, really help you.

Equally unhelpful is advice *against* alternative therapies that the woman who has breast cancer has decided to undergo. If she asks you for your opinion, then you're free to give it to her. But otherwise, you can best help her by listening to her and expressing your care for her.

*You are not responsible for determining why God allowed her to have cancer.* If she is asking that question herself, she probably wants to receive an answer directly from God, not from another human. If she seems to be truly looking to you for answers, you can share with her some ways that you yourself have experienced God in a time of crisis and perhaps a Scripture passage that helped you during that time. But be careful that your response doesn't come across as a solution to *her* problem. God expresses his love and care for each person in unique, personal ways, and you don't want to imply that whatever answers God gave you are the same answers that he would give her.

Realizing what you are not responsible for, in regard to helping a woman who has breast cancer, can free you to focus on what you can be responsible for. One task that you can be responsible for is to try to understand the woman's feelings. And that includes not minimizing, or trivializing, her cancer.

Frieda, for example, was diagnosed just a few months after a co-worker, Liz, had been treated for breast cancer. Unlike Liz, who had kept to herself and had avoided talking with her coworkers about her cancer, Frieda talked openly about her own cancer. But then something happened that troubled Frieda.

> Liz said to me one day, "People are saying that yours isn't as bad as mine was, and I said to them, 'Baloney! It's cancer. She's just handling it better than I did.'" I felt angry that people felt that way. I thought, *Please quit comparing me to Liz. Let me have my own disease.* I tried to understand why they were sort of pooh-poohing my experience with cancer. It may be that they'd been through it once and they knew that Liz came out OK; therefore, mine would be OK.

The flip side of trivializing a woman's cancer experience is calling more attention to it than she wants. Joan feels frustrated by people who ask her in a "whiny, pitying" voice, "Oh, Joan, how *arrrrre* you?" That kind of tone, Joan says, causes her to put up emotional walls. She responds with "OK" and then quickly ducks the spotlight by asking, "So how are things going with *you?*" She prefers that other people greet her in a way that sounds positive and normal, such as, "How are you doing, Joan?"

After the woman has been in treatment for a while, she might become tired of giving medical updates to all those who ask, especially to people who aren't involved in her daily life. Margaret discovered that she didn't appreciate so many people asking her—even without a pitying tone of voice—how she was doing. "I want to be honest and transparent, but I don't want to regurgitate all the truth," she says. "It makes me feel self-conscious, because I'm not used to talking about myself." Margaret doesn't mind giving medical details to a few friends, but from others she would rather hear "I'm so glad to see you" and other positive statements. For a woman who has cancer, a positive statement from others, rather than questions, relieves the pressure of having to decide whether to talk about her physical condition when she may not feel like talking about it.

Closely linked with trying to understand the woman's feelings is the importance of having the appropriate motive in helping her. If your motive is to help her and not to make yourself feel good, you're not as likely to feel hurt if she makes a special request such as "No cheese, please" when you offer to bring her a casserole and your specialty is lasagna.

Of course, it's appropriate to feel good when we do something to help someone else. But feeling good should be a byproduct, not the motive. Margaret tells of a woman who had found out that Margaret was ill and immediately wanted to do something for her. The woman persisted until Margaret asked her to purchase a special item that had been recommended to her. So the woman did. But the relationship became more uncomfortable and unhelpful to Margaret as soon as the woman arrived with the item. "She kept on talking, during her visit and as she was leaving, about how glad she was that she could do something for me—that it meant so much to her, because she felt so good," says Margaret, laughing. "For the person who is extremely self-serving, I can become an opportunity to make them feel better. That is my only function."

The kind of motivation that is helpful, Margaret says, is empathy. "There's a difference between a nervous desire to 'fix' this problem and a genuine desire to be involved with me in it." If you can express to the woman, in simple words, that you care about her and want to understand her feelings, that's probably the best gift you can give her. Beyond that, you might ask her what she needs from you. She may not have an answer immediately, but she'll probably appreciate the question.

### Helping the Woman's Family
If the woman who has breast cancer is your mother, daughter, wife, sister or other close family member, you are probably already aware of how powerfully a diagnosis of cancer can impact the entire family. And

you may be aware that your efforts to help your family member who has cancer have sometimes resulted in your own need for extra help. Although this section is directed primarily toward those who are outside the immediate family, it may help you to identify your own needs or those of other family members. If, however, you are not a family member, this section can help you find ways to help the family of a woman who has breast cancer.

One of the most helpful things that friends and relatives can do for the woman's family is to be alert to the ordinary needs of her family members. Jane's daughter, for example, was approaching her tenth birthday in the middle of Jane's chemotherapy treatments, and Jane, who believed that the tenth birthday should be a special one, felt bad that she had no energy to plan a celebration. But a friend of Jane's knew about the upcoming birthday and planned a party for Jane's daughter. On the day of the party, the friend positioned Jane in a comfortable chair where she could watch the children and participate in some of the activities. As someone who would have been uncomfortable asking for help, Jane greatly appreciated this perceptive and generous friend, who saw that something needed to be done and did it without being asked.

Family members of women who have cancer also have emotional needs that you might be able to meet. Janaha's story is a good example.

When Janaha was in high school and her mother had cancer, Janaha bathed her mother, helped her in the bathroom, prepared her food, helped to lift her from the bed to the wheelchair and back again each day, and took turns with her father sleeping in the living room, where her mother's hospital bed had been placed, so that her mother would never be alone. While Janaha was working hard to care for her mother, she not only was missing out on being with friends her own age but also was beginning to grieve the impending loss of her mother. And she needed but seldom had others to be with her as she grieved. That was her greatest difficulty.

I wish people would have more often shown concern toward me—*just me*—whether it was a phone call or whether it was someone coming to me and saying, "Can I take you somewhere?" I was home a lot, and there were times when I really needed to get away, so I'd go be by myself—

which was good, but I was already spending *enough* time in my thoughts. I felt like people would come over only to be with my mom, that she was the focal point of everything. And that was necessary; she was the one who had cancer. But I would get somewhat lost in the shadows. I felt like I could have used a little extra attention.

I think I needed a little more of someone saying, "How are *you?*" and "What can I do to help you?" At the time, I probably could have told them many, many ways they could have helped me. Someone to cry with, or someone to know what *I* was going through.

Janaha's peers were not an emotional support to her, perhaps because they "probably couldn't handle it," she says. Janaha felt alone, and her loneliness increased when one friend, with whom she had shared some of her feelings about her mother, said bluntly, "Get over it."

Janaha's situation is not unusual. She represents millions of teenage children, younger children, husbands, parents and siblings who are devastated by a family member's cancer. And if we care about the family members of the woman who has cancer, we are in a position to help them, even with simple gestures such as taking them out for coffee or a soda, engaging them in conversation about how their lives are different because of cancer, and remembering to pray for them.

### Helping a Woman Whose Diagnosis Is Terminal

When a woman you know has been told that her breast cancer is terminal, how do you respond? What can you say or do to show your care for her in light of this devastating news?

The suggestions discussed earlier for responding to any woman who has been diagnosed apply to this woman as well. She probably wants her friends to listen compassionately, to hug her, to reassure her of their care for her, to continue being involved in her life. And she still wants to be treated as a normal person as much as possible. But in addition, she wants other people to try to understand her perspective and her goals for the future, however short that future may be.

It's important not to assume that if her cancer has metastasized, or if her doctors don't expect her to survive, that *she* doesn't expect to survive. Often the woman herself is the last person to give up, and occasionally she surprises everyone by surviving. But no matter how bleak her future looks, as long as she has hopes for surviving, she needs to be supported in that hope by the people around her.

If she's made up her mind that she's going to live no matter what the doctors say, go along with her. Support her in her efforts to fight her cancer. If, however, she's trying to accept the likelihood of her impending death, it's vitally important, as it is with anyone diagnosed with cancer, to let her take the lead in your conversations with her. Listen carefully to whatever she says about God. Affirm any faith she has in God or in Christ. Whether she's a veteran Christian or a seeker who isn't sure what she believes, you may want to look for an opportunity to share with her whatever you yourself have experienced of God's love and faithfulness. Remember, though, that she is facing death and that unless you also are facing death, she may not trust your point of view.

Another difference in responding to a woman who is expected to die is that you and others who care about the woman are grieving over losing her, even while she's alive. That process is necessary and good; it prepares you somewhat for the actual loss. It's also good for the woman to know that you're grieving over losing her. If you've never expressed your appreciation of her and your care for her, it's not too late. She needs to know that you value her and that you will miss her.

If you have never personally faced probable death, particularly from a deadly disease, you have an opportunity to learn from a woman who is dying. Whether the woman has a strong faith or no faith, God can use your relationship with her to mature you and to draw you closer to him. Especially if you continue to be involved in the woman's life and in the lives of her family, you will never be the same, nor will you look at life in exactly the same way.

---

Here are some guidelines for responding to a woman who has been diagnosed with breast cancer:

■ Express your shock or sadness in hearing of her diagnosis. If you feel awkward and don't know what to say, remember that most women who share such news want only to hear that you feel shocked or saddened with them.

■ Give her your full attention as she talks further about her diagnosis. If she's telling you the news at a time that isn't convenient for you to respond in the way that you'd like, follow up with a phone call or a note.

■ Let her take the lead in discussing her breast cancer.

■ Avoid giving advice (unless she asks you for it) or asking her if she's been to see Dr. Fixit at The Cancer Clinic. She needs your understanding and your compassion, not your guidance.

■ If you want to encourage the woman by quoting a Scripture passage, choose verses that speak about God's love, comfort or mercy. Avoid any verses, such as Romans 8:28, that might explain the situation but do not encourage the sufferer.

■ Avoid telling her about someone else you know who has had breast cancer—unless it's you.

■ Tell her you'll pray for her (unless you know that she's uncomfortable with expressions of faith). And then be sure to do it.

---

**Here are a few suggestions for helping someone who is trying to feel normal in spite of her breast cancer:**

■ Talk with her about normal things: work, family, faith, church activities, hobbies, dreams for the future, the stock market, the outrageous salaries of celebrity athletes or whatever you would discuss with her if she were healthy.

■ Be aware, however, that because she's dealing with a life-threatening disease, she may not be in the mood for a lot of chit-chat. Be sensitive to how she responds to a topic you bring up. If she enthusiastically pursues it, then the topic is OK. But when you start hearing polite but brief responses from her, you might ask her if she's getting tired or if she would rather talk about something else.

■ Invite her to go with you on a specific outing—a movie, a shopping trip, a walk—or invite her out for lunch or over to your house for an evening. If she's not physically able to participate in the activity you suggest, ask her what kinds of things she can do, and suggest a date and a specific activity. Reassure her that the date is written in pencil, in case she needs to cancel at the last minute.

■ Invite her to participate in events as if she were completely healthy (she may be by now). But be prepared for her to decline. She needs to be given the choice to participate or not participate, without being pressured by anyone's expectations.

■ Remember that her family members are also trying to adjust to the ways that cancer has impacted their lives. Include them in outings, when appropriate. Plan an activity with one of them. Ask how she or he is feeling about this phase of the mother's (or wife's or sister's or daughter's) cancer experience, but talk about normal things as well.

---

# Appendix D

## RESOURCES

The resources listed here cover a wide range of cancer-related topics and are only a few of the many resources available. Inclusion does not imply endorsement, however.

**General Resources**
*Books and Periodicals*
Babcock, Elise NeeDell. *When Life Becomes Precious: A Guide for Loved Ones and Friends of Cancer Patients*. New York: Bantam, 1997.
*Coping with Cancer*. Bimonthly. Franklin, Tenn.: Media America. Phone: 615-790-2400. E-mail: Copingmag@aol.com
Kahane, Deborah Hobler. *No Less a Woman: Femininity, Sexuality and Breast Cancer*. Rev. 2nd ed. Alameda, Calif.: Hunter House, 1995.
Love, Susan, M.D., with Karen Lindsey. *Dr. Susan Love's Breast Book*. 2nd ed. Reading, Mass.: Addison-Wesley, 1995.
*Mamm: Women, Cancer and Community*. Bimonthly. New York: POZ Publishing.
McCarthy, Peggy, and Jo An Loren, eds. *Breast Cancer? Let Me Check My Schedule!* Boulder, Colo.: Westview Press, 1997.

Siegel, Bernie. *Love, Medicine and Miracles.* New York: Harper & Row, 1990.

Spiegel, David, M.D. *Living Beyond Limits: New Hope and Help for Facing Life-Threatening Illness.* New York: Times Books, 1993.

Stabiner, Karen. *To Dance with the Devil: The New War on Breast Cancer.* New York: Dell, 1997.

Steingraber, Sandra. *Living Downstream: A Scientist's Personal Investigation of Cancer and the Environment.* New York: Vintage Books, 1998.

Weiss, Marisa, M.D., and Ellen Weiss. *Living Beyond Breast Cancer.* New York: Times Books/Random House, 1997.

*Other General Resources*
American Cancer Society
1-800-ACS-2345

Bone Marrow Information
1-800-MARROW2

Cancer Information Service
1-800-4-CANCER

Hospice Education (for help with someone who is dying)
1-800-331-1620

National Asian Women's Health Organization
415-989-9747

National Cancer Institute
301-496-5583 (public inquiries)
For clinical trials: http://cancernet.nci.nih.gov
http://rex.nci.nih.gov
http://cancernet.nci.nih.gov

National Latina Health Organization
510-534-1362

National Women's Health Network
202-347-1140

National Y-ME (information, support and referrals to local chapters)
1-800-221-2141

The Susan G. Komen Breast Cancer Foundation
Occidental Tower
5005 LBJ Freeway, Suite 370
Dallas, Texas 75244
214-450-1777
Fax: 214-450-1710
Help line: 1-800-I'M AWARE (1-800-462-9273)

For up-to-date information on many cancers, available by fax:
CancerFax
301-402-5874

For information on adverse reactions to drug therapies:
1-800-FDA-1088 (1-800-332-1088)

*Rachel's Daughters: Searching for the Causes of Breast Cancer.* An Allie Light,
Irving Saraf and Nancy Evans film, 1997.

### Christian Resources
*Books*
Becton, Randy. *Everyday Strength: A Cancer Patient's Guide to Spiritual
Survival.* Grand Rapids, Mich.: Baker, 1989.
Bird, Rachel, and Juanita Ryan. *Together Living with Cancer: A Support
Group for People Who Have Been Diagnosed with Cancer and for Their
Loved Ones.* Leader's Manual. The Recovery Partnership, 1990. Can
be downloaded at no charge at www.christianrecovery.com
Buchanan, Sue. *I'm Alive and the Doctor's Dead!: Surviving Breast Cancer
with Your Sense of Humor and Your Sexuality Intact.* Grand Rapids,
Mich.: Zondervan, 1998. (Formerly published under the title *Love,
Laughter and a High Disregard for Statistics: Surviving Breast Cancer with
Your Sense of Humor and Your Sexuality Intact* [Nashville: Thomas
Nelson, 1994].)
Burkett, Larry, and Michael E. Taylor. *Hope When It Hurts: A Personal*

*Testimony of How to Deal with the Impact of Cancer.* Chicago: Moody Press, 1998.

Fintel, William A., M.D., and Gerard R. McDermott. *Dear God, It's Cancer: A Medical and Spiritual Guide for Patients and Their Families.* 2nd ed. Dallas: Word, 1997.

Hawkins, Don, Dan Koppersmith and Ginger Koppersmith. *When Cancer Comes: Healing for the Heart.* Chicago: Moody Press, 1993.

Hoek, Beatrice Hofman, with Melanie Jongsma. *Cancer Lives at Our House: Help for the Family.* Grand Rapids, Mich.: Baker, 1997.

Olmstead, Lois. *Breast Cancer and Me: A Humorous, Hope-Filled Story of a Breast Cancer Survivor.* Camp Hill, Penn.: Christian Publications, 1996.

*Other Christian Resources*
Dave Dravecky's Outreach of Hope
13840 Gleneagle Drive
Colorado Springs, CO 80921
719-481-3528
http://www.canpo.org/orgs/377.htm

"Surviving Breast Cancer." A two-cassette audiotape series featuring Dr. James Dobson and a panel of guests. Colorado Springs, Colo.: Focus on the Family, 1992.

*You are invited to contact Barbara Milligan about this book or about possible speaking engagements. You can e-mail her at bmilligan@ivpress.com or write her at InterVarsity Press, P.O. Box 1400, Downers Grove, IL 60515.*

# Notes

**Chapter 1: Turning to the God of Our Desperate Hope**
[1]National Cancer Institute, Surveillance Epidemiology and End Results (NCI SEER) program, "Cancer Statistics Review 1997." http://www.seer.ims.nci.nih.gov/index.html
[2]American Cancer Society, "Cancer Facts and Figures," 1998. http://www.cancer.org/frames.html

**Chapter 3: Responding to Feelings of Anger, Disappointment & Guilt**
[1]"What God Hath Promised," composed by William Runyan, lyrics by Annie Johnson Flint (Carol Stream, Ill.: Hope Publishing, 1919).

**Chapter 6: Facing Treatments & Their Side Effects**
[1]"The Flower That Shattered the Stone," Joe Henry and John Jarvis, Cherry Mountain Music, 1989.

**Chapter 7: Responding to Changes in Our Bodies**
[1]Wendy Shain, "Breast Cancer Surgeries and Psychosexual Sequaelae: Implications for Remediation," *Seminars in Oncology Nursing* 1, no. 3 (August 1985): 200-205, cited in Deborah Hobler Kahane, *No Less a Woman: Femininity, Sexuality and Breast Cancer,* 2nd ed. (Alameda, Calif.: Hunter House, 1995).

**Chapter 9: Keeping Our Relationships Intact**
[1]G. P. Murphy, W. L. Lawrence and R. E. Lenhard, eds., *Clinical Oncology* (Atlanta: American Cancer Society, 1995), pp. 198-219.

**Chapter 10: Grieving Our Losses**
[1]S. Lori Brown, Barbara G. Silverman and Wendie A. Berg, "Rupture of Silicone-Gel Breast Implants: Causes, Sequaelae, and Diagnosis." *The Lancet* 350 (November 22, 1997): 1531-37.

**Chapter 15: Renewing Our Hope**
[1]Barbara Ann Kipfer, *14,000 Things to Be Happy About* (New York: Workman Publishing, 1990)